Intraductal Biliary and Pancreatic Endoscopy

Guest Editor

PETER D. STEVENS, MD

GASTROINTESTINAL ENDOSCOPY CLINICS OF NORTH AMERICA

www.giendo.theclinics.com

Consulting Editor
CHARLES J. LIGHTDALE, MD

October 2009 • Volume 19 • Number 4

SAUNDERS an imprint of ELSEVIER, Inc.

W.B. SAUNDERS COMPANY
A Division of Elsevier Inc.

1600 John F. Kennedy Blvd. ● Suite 1800 ● Philadelphia, Pennsylvania 19103-2899

http://www.giendo.theclinics.com

GASTROINTESTINAL ENDOSCOPY CLINICS OF NORTH AMERICA Volume 19, Number 4
October 2009 ISSN 1052-5157, ISBN-13: 978-1-4377-1222-3, ISBN-10: 1-4377-1222-3

Editor: Kerry Holland

Gastrointestinal Endoscopy Clinics of North America (ISSN 1052-5157) is published quarterly by Elsevier Inc., 360 Park Avenue South, New York, NY 10010-1710. Months of issue are January, April, July, and October. Business and Editorial Offices: 1600 John F. Kennedy Blvd., Suite 1800, Philadelphia, PA, 19103-2899. Customer Service Office: 6277 Sea Harbor Drive, Orlando, FL 32887-4800. Periodicals postage paid at New York, NY and additional mailing offices. Subscription prices are $259.00 per year of US individuals $386.00 per year for US institutions, $133.00 per year for US students and residents, $286.00 per year for Canadian individuals, $471.00 per year for Canadian institutions, $362.00 per year for international individuals, $471.00 per year for international institutions, and $185.00 per year for Canadian and foreign students/residents. To receive student/resident rate, orders must be accompanied by name of affiliated institution, date of term, and the *signature* of program/residency coordinator on institution letterhead. Orders will be billed at individual rate until proof of status is received. Foreign air speed delivery is included in all *Clinics* subscription prices. All prices are subject to change without notice. **POSTMASTER:** Send address change to *Gastrointestinal Endoscopy Clinics of North America*, Elsevier Periodicals Customer Service, 11830 Westline Industrial Drive, St. Louis, MO 63146. **Customer Service: 1-800-654-2452 (US). From outside the United States, call 1-314-453-7041. Fax: 1-314-453-5170. E-mail: JournalsCustomerService-usa@elsevier.com (for print support) or JournalsOnline Support-usa@elsevier.com (for online support).**

Reprints. For copies of 100 or more, of articles in this publication, please contact the Commercial Reprints Department, Elsevier Inc., 360 Park Avenue South, New York, NY 10010-1710. Tel. (212) 633-3812; Fax: (212) 482-1935; E-mail: reprints@elsevier.com.

Gastrointestinal Endoscopy Clinics of North America is covered in *Excerpta Medica, MEDLINE/PubMed (Index Medicus), and MEDLINE/MEDLARS.*

Printed and bound by CPI Group (UK) Ltd, Croydon, CR0 4YY
Transferred to Digital Print 2011

Contributors

CONSULTING EDITOR

CHARLES J. LIGHTDALE, MD
Professor, Department of Medicine, Columbia University Medical Center, New York, New York

GUEST EDITOR

PETER D. STEVENS, MD
Associate Professor of Clinical Medicine, Division of Digestive and Liver Diseases, Columbia University College of Physicians and Surgeons; Director of Endoscopy, Columbia University Medical Center, New York Presbyterian Hospital, New York, New York

AUTHORS

JASON BRATCHER, MD
Therapeutic Endoscopy Fellow, Beth Israel Medical Center, New York, New York

KRISHNAVEL V. CHATHADI, MD
Assistant Professor of Medicine, Division of Gastroenterology and Hepatology, University of Colorado Denver; Therapeutic Endoscopist, Division of Gastroenterology, Denver Health Medical Center, Denver, Colorado

YANG K. CHEN, MD
Professor of Medicine, Division of Gastroenterology and Hepatology, University of Colorado Denver, Denver, Colorado; Director of Endoscopy/GI Practice, University of Colorado Hospital, Aurora, Colorado

GIOVANNI d'ADDAZIO, MD
Department of Medicine III – Gastroenterology, Interventional Endoscopy, St Bernward Academic Teaching Hospital, Hildesheim, Germany

GREGORY HABER, MD, MACG
Director, Division of Gastroenterology, Center for Advanced Therapeutic Endoscopy, Lenox Hill Hospital, New York, New York

JUERGEN HOCHBERGER, MD, PhD
Professor of Medicine and Chairman, Department of Medicine III – Gastroenterology, Interventional Endoscopy, St Bernward Academic Teaching Hospital, Hildesheim, Germany

TAKAO ITOI, MD
Department of Gastroenterology and Hepatology, Tokyo Medical University, Nishishinjuku, Shinjuku-ku, Tokyo, Japan

SHAHZAD IQBAL, MD
Instructor in Medicine, Division of Digestive and Liver Diseases, Department of Medicine, Columbia University College of Physicians and Surgeons, New York, New York

FRANKLIN KASMIN, MD
Medical Director, The Pancreas and Biliary Center, Saint Vincent's Hospital, New York, New York

RABI KUNDU, MD
Director of Endoscopy, Assistant Clinical Professor of Medicine, Division of Gastroenterology, University of California, San Francisco, Fresno, California

BENEDETTO MANGIAVILLANO, MD
Department of Gastroenterology and Gastrointestinal Endoscopy, San Paolo University Hospital, Milan, Italy

ALEXANDER MEINING, MD
Associate Professor of Medicine, Department of Medicine, II Medizinische Klinik, Klinikum rechts der Isar, Technical University of Munich, Müchen, Germany

HORST NEUHAUS, MD
Head, Department of Internal Medicine, Evangelisches Krankenhaus, Düsseldorf, Germany

SAM NOURANI, MS, MD
Private practice, Westlake Village, California

BRET T. PETERSEN, MD
Professor of Medicine, Division of Gastroenterology and Hepatology, Mayo Clinic, Rochester, Minnesota

DOUGLAS PLESKOW, MD
Co-Director of Endoscopy, Associate Clinical Professor of Medicine, Division of Gastroenterology, Beth Israel Deaconess Medical Center, Harvard Medical School, Boston, Massachusetts

DANIEL A. RINGOLD, MD
Instructor, Division of Gastroenterology and Hepatology, University of Colorado Denver, Aurora, Colorado

RAJ J. SHAH, MD
Associate Professor of Medicine and Director of Pancreaticobiliary Endoscopy Services, Division of Gastroenterology and Hepatology, University of Colorado Denver, Aurora, Colorado

PETER D. STEVENS, MD
Associate Professor of Clinical Medicine, Division of Digestive and Liver Diseases, Columbia University College of Physicians and Surgeons; Director of Endoscopy, Columbia University Medical Center, New York Presbyterian Hospital, New York, New York

PIER ALBERTO TESTONI, MD
Head, Division of Gastroenterology and Gastrointestinal Endoscopy, Vita-Salute San Raffaele University, Scientific Institute San Raffaele, Via Olgettina, Milan, Italy

Contents

Cholangiopancreatoscopy (CP) is a well-established modality for the direct visualization of intrahepatic biliary, extrahepatic biliary, and pancreatic ductal systems. The use of CP in the treatment of difficult biliary stones has become paramount when standard endoscopic retrograde cholangiopancreatography is ineffective. This article describes the available cholangioscopic devices and technical and clinical applications of cholangiopancreatoscopy. The efficacy and limitations of CP, as well as published comparative studies, are briefly reviewed.

The SpyGlass Direct Visualization System is a significant step forward in bringing optical visualization to the pancreatobiliary system by providing dedicated irrigation and therapeutic channels and 4-way steerability. Peroral cholangioscopy using the SpyGlass System may be safely performed by a single operator and provides reliable access to target sites for visual inspection and stone therapy using electrohydraulic lithotripsy or holmium laser lithotripsy. In addition, the SpyBite Biopsy Forceps has been shown to obtain adequate histologic tissue specimens reliably.

We summarized past and present results concerning the observation capability of cholangiopancratoscopy using chromoendoscopy, autofluorescence imaging (AFI), and narrow-band imaging (NBI). New generation peroral and percutaneous transhepatic video cholangiopancreatoscopes provide superior quality images. Pilot studies suggest that chromoendocholangioscopy using methylene blue or cholangioscopy using AFI can distinguish benign from malignant bile duct lesions. On the other hand, the NBI system enhances the imaging of certain features such as mucosal structures and microvessels in pancreatobiliary lesions. In patients with main-duct–type intraductal papillary mucinous neoplasm, peroral pancreatoscopy can be used to determine extent of tumor involvement. Although many technical hurdles still need to be overcome, image-enhanced cholangiopancratoscopy appears to be a promising modality to improve diagnostic accuracy of pancreatobiliary diseases, particularly in distinguishing benign from malignant lesions.

Establishing a tissue diagnosis in patients with suspected pancreaticobiliary malignancies remains challenging. Endoscopic retrograde cholangiopancreatography (ERCP)-based sampling methods have been reviewed in a previous issue of this journal but, unfortunately, the diagnostic yield continues to be inadequate in a significant minority of patients. The availability and image quality of cholangioscopy and pancreatoscopy have advanced in the last few years and our ability to make a diagnosis on imaging alone is improving. However, a definitive diagnosis requires tissue; cholangiopancreatoscopy allows targeted biopsies of the epithelium of the biliary and pancreatic ducts. This article reviews the evidence that cholangioscopy- and pancreatoscopy-guided biopsies improves diagnostic yield over ERCP-based tissue sampling techniques.

Cholangioscopy is gaining renewed interest and gradually expanded use as a result of recent technical improvements in endoscopes and accessories, coupled with shortcomings in the accuracy of currently available techniques for biliary sampling and diagnosis. Challenging clinical dilemmas that may benefit from its application include early diagnosis of cholangiocarcinoma in the setting of primary sclerosing cholangitis, early identification of biliary infection or ischemia following orthotopic liver transplantation, and selective duct access with wires and other devices during therapeutic endoscopic retrograde cholangiopancreatography. Preliminary data suggest that cholangioscopy has significant utility in assessment and management of primary sclerosing cholangitis. Applications in post-transplant patients and for selective duct access remain minimally defined and used.

In more than 90% of choledocholithiasis cases, endoscopic retrograde cholangiopancreatography with sphincterotomy and stone extraction are successful therapeutic options for clearance of the bile duct with the use of a stone retrieval balloon or basket. However, these techniques fail in a small percentage of patients with biliary stones, and advanced techniques for fragmentation must be used. Intraductal shock wave lithotripsy offers the endoscopist a therapeutic option that may be effective despite the difficulties of a large, impacted stone that cannot be captured by a basket, or a stricture that prohibits delivery of a stone beyond it. This article reviews the use of electrohydraulic lithotripsy and laser lithotripsy in the clinical setting.

with confocal miniprobes further miniaturized to such an extent to enable their use even via the instrumentation channel of cholangioscopes. The current data available suggest that this new technology represents a promising approach for further differentiation of strictures and stenosis in the biliary, and perhaps also pancreatic system. Nevertheless, those results are based on a limited number of patients; further studies involving more patients examined at various centers are necessary and already under way to prove the true clinical importance of this new imaging modality.

Optical coherence tomography (OCT) is an optical imaging modality introduced in 1991 that performs high-resolution, cross-sectional, subsurface tomographic imaging of the microstructure in materials and biologic systems by measuring backscattered or backreflected infrared light. OCT has been used for biomedical applications where many factors affect the feasibility and effectiveness of any imaging technique. The highly scattering and absorbing living tissues greatly limit the application of optical imaging modalities. In the last decade, OCT technology has evolved from an experimental laboratory tool to a new diagnostic imaging modality with a wide spectrum of clinical applications in medical practice, including the gastrointestinal (GI) tract and pancreaticobiliary ductal system.

THE CLINICS ARE NOW AVAILABLE ONLINE!

Access your subscription at:
www.theclinics.com

Foreword

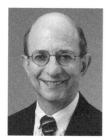

Charles J. Lightdale, MD
Consulting Editor

Just when it seemed that all endoscopic frontiers had been crossed, intraductal biliary and pancreatic endoscopy or cholangiopancreatoscopy has emerged as a robust new area for exploration in gastrointestinal endoscopy. Although endoscopic retrograde cholangiopancreatography (ERCP) combines endoscopy with fluoroscopy and has resulted in remarkable progress in the management of diseases affecting the bile and pancreas ducts, it remains a hybrid procedure, providing indirect radiographic images. With the development of ever-thinner endoscopes, first fiberoptic and now tiny, powerful charge-coupled device chip video, real-time, high-quality visual imaging of the ducts via oral intubation of the papilla of Vater has become a reality.

Intraductal biliary and pancreatic endoscopy offers tremendous opportunities for diagnosis and therapy. A through-the-scope channel allows visually guided biopsy, lithotripsy, and stone removal. New optical methods can be applied for more precise and detailed analysis of tissue within the ducts. Areas of active research involve the identification of premalignant lesions and the earliest stage cancers involving the ducts and treatment with minimally invasive endoscopic methods.

Cholangiopancreatoscopy requires considerable skill and experience with ERCP. I was introduced to this technique by Dr Peter D. Stevens, a colleague at New York–Presbyterian Hospital/Columbia University Medical Center. I know Pete to be one of the most skilled gastrointestinal endoscopists on the planet, who has done pioneering research in interventional endoscopy, but I was still amazed the first time I watched him scope the bile duct through a small papillotomy. I immediately determined to ask him if he would be guest editor for an issue of the *Gastrointestinal Endoscopy Clinics of North America* on "Intraductal Biliary and Pancreatic Endoscopy." He has assembled an

Gastrointest Endoscopy Clin N Am 19 (2009) xi–xii
doi:10.1016/j.giec.2009.09.002
giendo.theclinics.com
1052-5157/09/$ – see front matter © 2009 Elsevier Inc. All rights reserved.

extraordinary group of experts to cover all aspects of this endoscopic frontier, and the result is a landmark issue of the *Clinics*. If you are doing ERCP, this is a must-read volume.

Charles J. Lightdale, MD
Department of Medicine
Columbia University Medical Center
161 Fort Washington Avenue, Room 812
New York, NY 10032, USA

E-mail address:
CJL18@columbia.edu

Preface

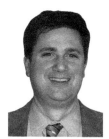

Peter D. Stevens, MD
Guest Editor

Contrast radiography has given way to endoscopy for the evaluation of the upper gastrointestinal tract, the small bowel, and the colon. The pancreaticobiliary ductal system has remained the one area in which gastroenterologists depend heavily on contrast-enhanced fluoroscopy. The concept of entering the ducts with an endoscope is certainly not new; peroral cholangiopancreatoscopy has been possible for decades. The discipline has been enjoying a resurgence of interest, however, as the equipment has become increasingly miniaturized, maneuverable, and manageable. Furthermore, new diagnostic technologies and therapeutic accessories have been developed for intraductal applications that have widely expanded capabilities. This issue of *Gastrointestinal Endoscopy Clinics of North America* focuses on these advances in intraductal endoscopy that are allowing exploration of one of the last endoscopic frontiers.

The first article, by Drs Nourani and Haber, gives a comprehensive overview of the technical aspects of and clinical applications for cholangiopancreatoscopy. They review the details of currently available cholangioscopes and current clinical applications with many pearls of endoscopic wisdom useful to endoscopists of all levels. In the second article, Drs Chathadi and Chen expand on the technical aspects of the only semidisposable cholangioscopic system, the SpyGlass Direct Visualization System. They review the system in detail and discuss the preclinical and clinical data that are accumulating in addition to highlighting some potentially useful novel applications. In the third article, Drs Itoi, Neuhaus, and Chen illustrate the potential of image-enhanced cholangiopancreatoscopy. In the fourth article, Dr Iqbal and I review the power of targeted biopsies to augment intraductal imaging.

Leading off the therapeutic articles, Dr Petersen tackles the difficult area of cholangioscopy in special patients and situations. His experience with primary sclerosing cholangitis and post–liver transplant patients makes him especially suited for this review. Fellow New Yorkers, Drs Kasmin and Bratcher, cover one of the most useful applications of intraductal endoscopy: lithotripsy of large bile duct stones. Moving to the pancreatic duct specifically, Drs Hochberger and D'Addazio explore the field of

Gastrointest Endoscopy Clin N Am 19 (2009) xiii–xiv
doi:10.1016/j.giec.2009.09.003
1052-5157/09/$ – see front matter © 2009 Elsevier Inc. All rights reserved.

intraductal tumor treatment. Dr Ringold and Shah review the use of intraductal endoscopy for intraductal papillary mucinous neoplasms and strictures.

Finally, three advanced areas of intraductal imaging are addressed: Drs Kundu and Pleskow discuss intraductal ultrasound, Dr Meining discusses confocal endomicroscopy, and Drs Testoni and Mangiavillano provide insights into optical coherence tomography.

I would like to thank all of the authors for taking the time from their busy clinical and academic workload to produce the articles for this issue. I would also like to thank Dr Charles Lightdale for the wonderful opportunity to guest edit this issue and bring all of these intraductal technologies together in a single volume. I remember that he asked me initially if I thought there would be enough material for an entire issue, and, as you read through this volume, I think you will agree that there is. Finally I would like to thank Kerry Holland and her staff at Elsevier, without whose hard work this issue would have never been possible.

Peter D. Stevens, MD
Department of Medicine
Columbia University Medical Center
New York, NY, USA

E-mail address:
pds5@columbia.edu

Cholangiopancreatoscopy: A Comprehensive Review

Sam Nourani, MS, MD[a],*, Gregory Haber, MD, MACG[b]

KEYWORDS

- Choledochoscopy • Cholangioscopy
- Cholangiopancreatoscopy • Pancreatoscopy
- Intrahepatic biliary strictures • Percutaneous

Cholangiopancreatoscopy (CP) is performed with the use of miniature endoscopes to directly visualize the ducts of the biliary and pancreatic systems. Cholangioscopy was first used intraoperatively during open bile duct exploration for localization of stones,[1] after which the cholangioscope was used postoperatively through an established T-tube tract for stone detection, intraductal lithotripsy, and biopsy.[2,3] CP has since been developed for further applications such as percutaneous transhepatic cholangiography (PTCS),[4] retrograde cholangiography,[5] and retrograde pancreatography[6] to localize, and diagnose disorders, acquire tissue, remove stones with or without intraductal lithotripsy, ablate tumors, and place wires. Early retrograde CP was performed with a specially designed large 5.5-mm channel duodenoscope to accommodate the 4.5-mm cholangioscope, the so-called mother-daughter system.[6–9] Optical research and endoscopic design has allowed the development of cholangioscopes capable of passing through the working channel of a standard therapeutic duodenoscope.[10]

CHOLANGIOSCOPIC DEVICES

In the United States there are various fiberoptic cholangoscopes on the market. Olympus and Pentax offer reusable fiberoptic cholangioscopes, whereas Boston Scientific offers the only semidisposable fiberoptic cholangioscope (**Table 1**).[11] The peroral route uses small cholangioscopes (2.6, 2.8, 3.1, and 3.4 mm) with longer working channel lengths (187, 190, and 200 cm). The accessory channel for the 2.6- and 2.8-mm cholangioscopes is 0.75-mm, which allows for a 0.025-in guide wire. The 3.1-, 3.4-, and a special order 2.8-mm cholangioscope has a 1.2-mm accessory channel that allows for a 0.035-in guide wire, biopsy forceps, or a 1.9F to 3F electrohydraulic lithotripsy (EHL) fiber.

All of these cholangioscopes require a therapeutic duodenoscope with a 4.2-mm working channel to access the major papilla (**Fig. 1**). To pass these cholangioscopes into the ampulla, a sphincterotomy is usually necessary. However, there are situations

[a] 686 Triunfo Canyon Road, Westlake Village, CA 91361, USA
[b] Division of Gastroenterology, Center for Advanced Therapeutic Endoscopy, Lenox Hill Hospital, 100 East 77th St, NY 10075, USA
* Corresponding author.
E-mail address: samnourani@gmail.com (S. Nourani).

Gastrointest Endoscopy Clin N Am 19 (2009) 527–543
doi:10.1016/j.giec.2009.07.003
1052-5157/09/$ – see front matter © 2009 Elsevier Inc. All rights reserved.

Table 1
Cholangioscopes

Company	Model	Field of View (degrees)	Depth of Field (mm)	Distal Diameter (mm)	Accessory Channel (mm)	Angulation Up/Down (Degrees)	Angulation Right/Left (Degrees)	Per Oral	Working Length (cm)
Olympus, Center Valley, PA	CHF-BP30	90	1–50	3.4	1.2	160/130	n/a	Yes	187
	CHF-B160	90	1–30	3.4	1.2	90/90	n/a	Yes	200
	CHF-BP160	90	1–30	2.6	0.5	90/90	n/a	Yes	200
	XCHF-BP160F	90	2–50	2.8	1.2	70/70	n/a	Yes	200
Pentax, Orangeburg, NY	FCP-8P	90	1–50	2.8	0.75	90/90	n/a	Yes	190
	FCP-9P	90	1–50	3.1	1.2	90/90	n/a	Yes	190
Boston Scientific, Marlboro, MA	Spyglass probe (reusable)	70	1–50	0.81	n/a	n/a	n/a	Yes	300
	Spyscope (single use)	n/a	n/a	3.4	1.2/0.6/ 0.6/0.9[a]	90/90	90/90	Yes	230

Abbreviation: n/a, not available.
[a] Indicates diameter in millimeters for accessory channel, irrigation lumen, irrigation lumen, and optical probe lumen, respectively.

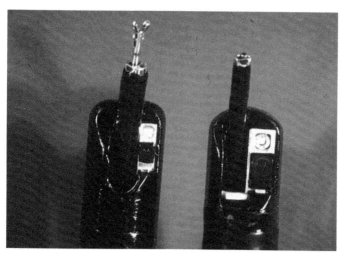

Fig. 1. Mother-daughter scopes.

in which a daughter scope is not necessary, when a gastroscope (5.9 and 8.8 mm outer diameter [OD])[12,13] can be used instead for direct inspection of the bile duct. For percutaneous and intraoperative approaches a larger (4.8, 4.9, and 6.0 mm) cholangioscope with a shorter (35, 38, 45, and 70 cm) working length, and a larger (2.0, 2.2, and 2.6 mm) accessory channel is available that accommodates more therapeutic tools: retrieval forceps, baskets, and larger intraductal lithotripsy fibers.[11]

The control area of the reusable cholangioscopes have a lever for a 2-way up/down tip deflection, and buttons for air/water and suction channels. The core of the cholangioscope consists of a bundle of glass fibers that transmits the image from the tip of the endoscope to the eyepiece, an objective lens system at the tip of the endoscope, a light guide for illumination, angulation wires for tip deflection, an air/water nozzle to keep the lens clear, and a single instrument channel. The cholangioscopes differ by tip deflection angle, OD, working channel size, field of view, and available accessories (see **Table 1**). For percutaneous and intraoperative cholangioscopy, the scopes have a larger OD and are capable of having more optical fibers, improving illumination, image resolution, and field of vision.[11]

The Boston Scientific Spyscope device is a semidisposable device with 2 main components: a flexible delivery catheter and a handle. The device is intended to be used to guide both an optical probe and accessory devices. This device has 4-way tip deflection with a locking lever to lock the distal tip in position. Three ports are available for use: an irrigation port that feeds into two 0.6-m channels, an optical probe port, and a 1.2-mm accessory channel. The optical probe is composed of a polyamide sheath, which encloses a collection of light fibers that surround optical fiber bundles producing 6000-pixel resolution.

As discussed earlier, the cholangioscopes used in clinical practice are primarily fiberoptic-based technology. However, a 3.4- and 5.3-mm video cholangioscope, an ultraminiature (2.6 mm with a 0.5-mm working channel) video cholangioscope using charge-coupled device (CCD) technology, and a narrow-band imaging system incorporated into a video cholangioscope are investigational, and have limited commercial availability.[14–17] The video cholangioscopes, however, have better image quality due to the CCD technology positioned at the distal end of the endoscope, and have a lighter control area because of the absence of the bulky fiber optic bundles.[11] A new technology in development, scanning single-fiber endoscopy, can produce high-quality images using catheter-style endoscopes as small as 1 mm in diameter.[18,19]

TECHNICAL APPLICATIONS
Peroral Cholangioscopy

The peroral approach using the reusable cholangioscope is ideally a 2-operator procedure. However, a single operator can perform both roles with a specially de-signed external cholangioscope fixation device.[20] Alternatively, a nurse or technician can take the same role as the fixation device, with no need for robotic innovation for simple adjustments in the manipulation of the "baby or daughter scope." Before intro-ducing the cholangioscope, the ampulla and pancreaticobiliary system should be delineated with cholangiopancreatography to determine the feasibility of introducing and advancing a small caliber scope into the duct system. Unless an ultrathin, wire-guided scope is used, it will be necessary to perform a sphincterotomy or stricture dilation if needed. Introduction of the daughter scope can be performed "freehand" by directing the tip through the papilla with judicious use of the elevator to avoid damage from compression of the elevator, especially with the newly designed "V" groove, located on the elevator of the duodenoscope. The up-and-down deflection plane of the choledochoscope must match that of the elevator of the duodenoscope to facilitate ductal insertion.

The alternative introduction method is the wire-guided introduction. A long 450-cm wire is introduced into the duct and then back-loaded into the channel of the daughter scope before introducing the daughter scope into the duodenoscope. Wire guidance reduces the need for elevator use during cannulation, which will reduce the likelihood of damage that might cause leaks in the bending portion of the cholangioscope. Once the scope is advanced to the target lesion, the guide wire is removed to allow use of the accessory channel for irrigation and introduction of devices.

Lubricating the duodenoscope accessory channel or the distal end of the cholangio-scope will allow easier endoscopic passage. The guide wire is especially useful in those instances when it is necessary to move the tip of the duodenoscope away from the papilla to accommodate the introduction of the daughter scope, resulting in a less than optimal view of the papilla. In such cases, simultaneous use of the guide wire along with fluoroscopic guidance will allow introduction of the cholangioscope and then repositioning of the mother scope. The best approach usually for daughter scope introduction is to have the duodenoscope tip as close to the papilla as possible, to reduce the angulation at which the cholangioscope is introduced into the duct. The cholangioscope's controls should be kept in the unlocked position when the scope is advanced past the papilla, or directional control can be guided by the fluoroscopic road map. When performing cholangioscopy with 2 operators, the one controlling the up/down tip deflection is also responsible for introduction of biopsy forceps for tissue sampling or intraductal lithotripsor for stone fragmentation. Alternatively, this can be performed by a single operator, whereby the control area of the cholangio-scope is placed into an opening on a specially designed breastplate secured onto the endoscopist, or held by an assistant standing beside the endoscopist.[11,20]

The optical probe of the semidisposable cholangioscopic device is first preloaded into the access catheter and advanced to within a few millimeters of the catheter's bending portion, to avoid potential damage during passage across the duodeno-scope's elevator. The control area is attached to the barrel of the duodenoscope, below the working channel; it is then inserted into the working channel of the duodenoscope with or without the use of a guide wire. Once ampullary cannulation is achieved, the optical probe is advanced beyond the catheter's tip for intraductal evaluation. The 4-way tip is maneuvered by the endoscopist with steering dials that may be locked in a position to allow for tissue biopsy or EHL. Irrigation is performed through a separate channel or through the accessory channel. If a guide wire or EHL fiber is present, a specialized Y-adapter must be placed for coaxial irrigation for debris dislodgement.

Percutaneous Cholangioscopy

Percutaneous cholangioscopy can be performed by a gastroenterologist or interventional radiologist with an assistant for guide wire, biopsy forceps, or EHL fiber. The route for choledochoscopy can occur through an operatively placed T-tube tract or by percutaneous transhepatic biliary drainage (PTBD) (**Fig. 2**).[21] The drawback of the T-tube is that the tract must be formed 3 to 5 weeks before it can be used for the passage of instruments. Due to the inherent time delay there are patient management issues, not to mention the resources and risks associated with extended anesthesia and surgery to establish the T-tube access.[22] For more detailed description regarding operative T-tube placement, the reader is referred to the surgical literature.

For PTBD, patients should receive antibiotic prophylaxis to prevent cholangitis, typically a second-generation cephalosporin administered an hour before the procedure.[23,24] The first step in PTBD is to establish percutaneous access to the ducts of choice in the liver. In North America, this is usually done by an interventional radiologist, whereas in many countries in Europe a gastroenterologist with appropriate training can perform this procedure. After access to the duct with cholangiography, a 7F to 8F pigtail catheter is advanced into the biliary ducts and down to the duodenum under fluoroscopic guidance. The tract is then allowed to mature over 2 to 4 weeks. However, after several days the tract is sequentially dilated to allow introduction of a large 16F diameter catheter to maximize the tract diameter before

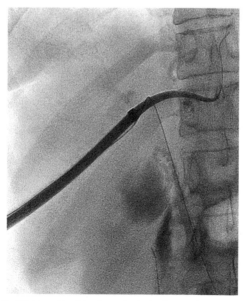

Fig. 2. Dilation of percutaneous tract before choledochoscopy.

preprocedure dilation, which is the final step before introduction of the cholangio-scope and accessories.[25] The waiting period is required for stabilization and matura-tion of the wall of the dilated tract, to prevent traversal into the peritoneal cavity when the cholangioscope is introduced directly through the skin.

When the clinical situation does not allow for a delayed approach, it is necessary to use a sheath between the skin and the liver for choledochoscope introduction. Plastic peel-away sheaths (Cook Inc) or a metallic sheath (Olympus Inc) are avail-able that were designed for a percutaneous nephroscope. The sheaths are advanced over tapered bougies, which dilate the tract up to the necessary diameter. As most choledochoscopes have an OD of 5 mm, the sheath size required must provide an internal diameter of at least 5.2 mm, which usually necessitates a sheath of 20F.[23]

In patients with common bile duct (CBD) stones a single percutaneous tract can be created in the right or left lobe, but the right access route is typically preferred as it is technically easier to access, with less radiation exposure, and is less bothersome for the patient.[23] The selection of the puncture site is very important and depends on the stone locations (left approach for stones on the right side and right approach for stones on the left side). When CBD stones are found, the left approach is the ideal choice because it is easier to pass the scope from the left intrahepatic duct either toward the right side or down through the CBD, but it is often difficult to pass the scope from the right to the left (**Fig. 3**).[26] However, in some patients with stones in both lobes, multiple tracts, typically 2 to 3, may be necessary.[23]

The same approach also applies regarding tract placement for mapping of cholan-giocarcinoma.[27] Biopsy mapping under percutaneous cholangioscopy guidance is useful in patients with resectable bile duct cancer because it often demonstrates longitudinal tumor extension along the bile duct.[28] As previously reported, when endoscopic retrograde cholangiopancreatography (ERCP) findings show a tumor with a collapsed edge there is an increased incidence of longitudinal spread, and preoperative mapping with biopsies is essential to determine a suitable surgical line of resection. The extension of cholangiocarcinoma in the submucosa and along perineural planes makes it difficult to assess the margins of the tumor with cholangi-ography or cross-sectional imaging. As distinct vascular markings and subtle surface changes can only be appreciated under direct cholangioscopic inspection, many surgeons prefer to perform percutaneous cholangioscopy before major liver resec-tion in an attempt to improve an R0 resection margin.

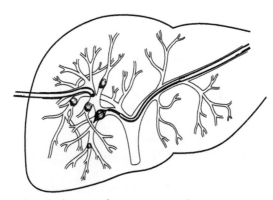

Fig. 3. Percutaneous choledochoscopy for stone extraction.

The visualization and direct treatment of large intraductal stones with EHL is one of the foremost therapeutic breakthroughs of CP. The ability to directly visualize the stone within the duct is mandatory when using EHL to avoid bile duct injury (**Fig. 4**). The EHL is a bipolar coaxial electrode that discharges a rapid series of sparks at the electrode tip. When the electrode tip is placed in an electrolyte solution and discharged, the high-voltage sparks cause an explosive evaporation and sudden expansion of the surrounding fluid that initiates the creation of hydraulic shock waves. When a shock wave travels through liquid, its energy is absorbed by an abrupt increase in acoustic resistance such as provided by a stone. Absorption of shock wave energy within the stone leads to a buildup of pressure gradients that allow for shear forces to eventually cause fragmentation (**Fig. 5**).[29]

Irrigation is a critical component of lithotripsy not only to provide a medium for propagation of shock waves but also to allow clear visualization. Mucoid material is usually present, which obscures the field of view, and as the choledochoscopes have a tiny water channel, additional irrigation is mandatory. Furthermore, once stone fragmentation begins there is a cloud of stone debris that fills the field of view. There are 2 methods to achieve irrigation, either through the operating channel of the cholangioscope or via an external nasobiliary drain. The Spyscope system has a separate channel for irrigation built into the scope. Coaxial irrigation alongside an EHL probe in the accessory channel is effective only with a minimal channel diameter of 1.2 mm; if any smaller, coaxial flow is ineffectual. The saline flow can be controlled in several ways. There are dedicated water pumps, syringe systems that require an assistant to push the saline on demand, or gravity-dependent flow from an intravenous bag that requires a compression sleeve to be of any value.

The tip of the EHL fiber should protrude 2 to 4 mm from the scope and be positioned en face with the stone, thereby reducing the risk of inadvertent ductal contact. The probe should be gently applied to the stone but not firmly, as there must be a putative space to allow formation of the hydraulic shock wave. Energy may then be delivered by activating the generator (**Fig. 6**) via a foot pedal.[29] It has been found that the bile duct wall cannot be damaged at any power setting with the probe tip within 1 mm from the duct. When the probe was placed in direct contact with the duct wall the spark energy "vaporized" the wall.[30]

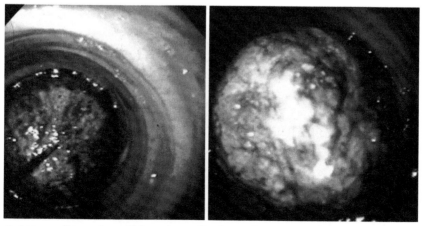

Fig. 4. Large gallstone in small bowel, manifesting as Bouveret syndrome, before EHL.

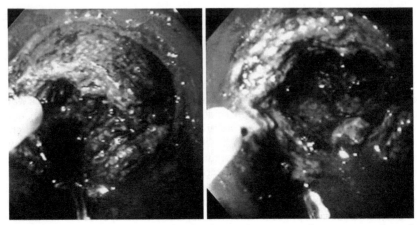

Fig. 5. EHL of large gallstone within the duodenum (treatment of Bouveret syndrome).

CLINICAL APPLICATIONS

When ERCP was introduced in 1970 followed by endoscopic sphincterotomy in 1974, there was a quantum advance in the diagnosis and treatment of pancreatobiliary disorders.[31] However, in some instances direct endoscopic visualization of the biliary and pancreatic ducts may be needed for definitive pathologic diagnosis or to provide therapeutic interventions.

Experience with choledochoscopy was initially reported by Kawai and colleagues[32] in 1976, followed by several reports from Japan and Europe. Enthusiasm for this technology declined for 2 reasons: first, because of the simultaneous improvements in noninvasive imaging techniques such as ultrasound and computed tomography and second, because of the extreme fragility and cost of the initially available instruments. However, almost 40 years of experience with CP has shown that there are certain pancreatobiliary disorders in which ERCP alone may not be adequate.[33] One of the key therapeutic benefits of CP is the capacity to directly visualize and treat large intraductal stones, and CP has been used to evaluate equivocal fluoroscopy findings during ERCP, PTCS, and intraoperative cholangiography (IOC). Because direct visualization

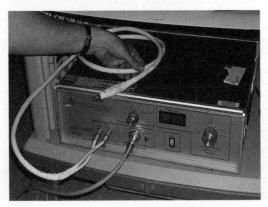

Fig. 6. EHL generator.

is not possible with ERCP, intraductal tumors may mimic large stones, benign-appearing biliary strictures may be malignant (**Fig. 7**), and strictures thought to be malignant may be benign. With CP the rate of these false positives and false negatives can be reduced.[21]

Diagnostic applications have been reported for characterizing strictures and determining the morphologic features and extent of malignancies: cholangiocarcinoma, intraductal papillary mucinous neoplasia, and intraductal tubular neoplasia. Detecting occult stones and cholangiocarcinoma in patients with primary sclerosing cholangitis (PSC), and use after orthotopic liver transplant (OLT) when an opportunistic infection may be a possible cause of a biliary stricture or ulcer, are additional diagnostic uses for CP.

Diagnostic applications of CP
- Intraductal stone visualization
- Evaluation of equivocal fluoroscopic findings of ERCP, PTCS, or IOC
- Defining morphology and extent of cholangiocarcinoma, intraductal papillary mucinous neoplasm (IPMN), intraductal tubular neoplasm
- Detection of occult stones or cholangiocarcinoma in PSC
- Hemobilia of unknown etiology
- Evaluation of biliary strictures after OLT

Therapeutic applications include tissue sampling, removal of stones in conjunction with EHL, traversing difficult strictures that cannot be traversed using standard techniques, diagnosis, and treatment of hemobilia of unknown etiology, directed application of laser energy with quartz fibers for photodynamic therapy, and treatment of

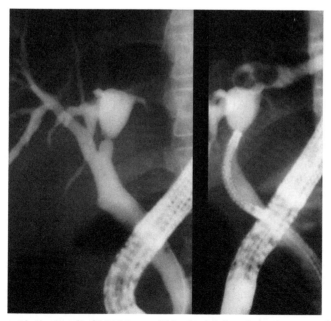

Fig. 7. Fluoroscopic images. (*Left*) Stricture within the left intrahepatic system. (*Right*) Choledochoscopy of the left intrahepatic system with intrahepatic stones upstream from a stricture.

occluded self-expandable metallic stents. Direct visualization of the biliary ducts allows for recognition of unsuspected abnormalities and endoscopically guided tissue sampling or therapy.

Therapeutic applications of CP
    EHL
    Tissue sampling
    Palliative therapy for biliary malignancies
    Facilitation of selective guide-wire access to the gallbladder or intrahepatic ducts

On occasion, the peroral route may not be feasible or fails. This failure may occur because of difficulties accessing the papilla; duodenal obstruction by malignancy, or with changes in intestinal anatomy (eg, Billroth II, Roux-en-Y anastomosis), with ductal location (eg, beyond the hilum or above strictures), in the setting of inaccessible intrahepatic stones or difficult-to-treat CBD stones,[4,26] or to assess the upstream spread of cholangiocarcinoma.[27] In these settings percutaneous cholangioscopy is preferable.

Intraoperative cholangioscopy is used during open or laparoscopic bile duct exploration to assess ductal patency and localize bile duct stones.[34–37] There are limited reports of intraoperative pancreatoscopy for treatment of stones in the pancreatic duct[38] or to localize an IPMN for resection.[39]

EFFICACY

Peroral cholangioscopy with EHL will allow complete removal of complicated choledocholithiasis, defined as those that failed ERCP and had stones larger than 2 cm; stones above a narrow duct segment; impacted stones; or stones lodged in the cystic duct. In the largest series to date, 111 patients who had on average 2 failed ERCPs per patient with failed stone extraction from the extrahepatic biliary system revealed that 96% of patients had successful fragmentation with EHL, with 76% requiring a single session. Fragmentation failures were due to targeting issues and stone density. Final stone clearance was achieved in 90% of patients.[9] A second series of 32 patients had an average of 3.3 failed ERCPs per patient for intrahepatic and extrahepatic stone disease. Cholangioscopy identified additional stones not seen at ERCP in 28% of patients. On average, 1.4 lithotripsy sessions achieved complete stone clearance in 81% of patients. Follow-up on 88% of patients at mean 29 months revealed 18% stone recurrence.[8] Peroral cholangioscopy was also shown to be effective in 64% of patients with hepatolithiasis when used in combination with extracorporeal shock wave lithotripsy (ESWL).[40] However, a 20% rate of stone recurrence in patients with intrahepatic stones or PSC is to be expected.[8,41] A percutaneous or surgical approach could become warranted in settings of decreased duct clearance rates: surgically altered anatomy, downstream strictures, acute intrahepatic ductal angulation, and impacted stones.

For intrahepatic stones inaccessible to coupled peroral cholangioscopy and EHL, percutaneous cholangioscopy and EHL achieves duct clearance in up to 85% of patients.[26,42] However, in the presence of intrahepatic strictures or retained occult stone fragments, recurrence rates of stones or cholangitis may reach up to 50%. In these series of cases, EHL was used in conjunction with cholangioscopy less than 10% of the time because large stones upstream of intrahepatic strictures were removed percutaneously with a retrieval basket.

In the context of biliary malignancy, cholangioscopy guides tissue sampling by identifying "tumor vessels," that is, vascular and mucosal signs of malignancy. These signs include irregular mucosa, intense neovascularization (**Fig. 8**), intraductal nodules (**Fig. 9**), infiltrative or ulcerated strictures (**Figs. 10** and **11**), and papillary (**Fig. 12**) or villous mucosal projections.[22] The sensitivity in detecting cholangiocarcinoma in a cohort of patients with known cancer was 100% for the polypoid type, 95% for the stenotic type, and 100% when a tumor vessel pattern was appreciated. However, detection was only 60% for pancreatic cancer that obstructed the bile duct.[27] The importance of proper tissue sampling needs emphasizing, because tissue sampling from the margins and not from within strictures improved the histologic diagnosis rate of stenotic-type cholangiocarcinoma from 70% to 100%.[27] When combining cholangioscopic evidence of tumor vessel with percutaneous biopsy, the sensitivity of cancer diagnosis increased from 61% to 96% compared with cholangioscopy alone.[43] For the treatment of patients with pancreatic duct stones, 2 small case series showed complete main duct clearance rates of 100% with intraoperative EHL followed by decompressive surgery ($n = 10$)[44] compared with a clearance rate of only 50% with peroral pancreatoscopy with EHL and ESWL ($n = 6$).[45] A majority of patients in both series had symptom improvement, with complete or partial clearance. A larger study of 115 patients that evaluated pancreatic strictures with a minimum 2-year follow-up found that pancreatoscopy detected 63% of pancreatic cancers, 80% of benign strictures, and 95% of IPMN lesions.[46] The visual clues used to assess neoplasia included tumor vessel (as described earlier), friability, coarse mucosa, subepithelial protrusion, and papillary projections.[46,47] The visual clues to delineate malignant from benign IPMN include endoscopic evidence, fish egg–like, villous, and prominent mucosal protrusions with a sensitivity and specificity of 68% and 87%, respectively. However, lower sensitivities at malignant detection were appreciated for branch duct IPMN compared with main duct IPMN.

Cholangioscopic guide: signs of malignancy
    Irregular mucosa
    Intense neovascularization
    Intraductal nodules

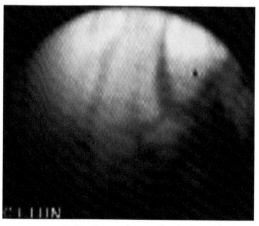

Fig. 8. Pancreatoscopy: neovascularization at base of tubular neoplasm.

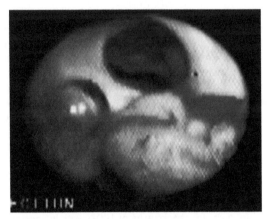

Fig. 9. Pancreatoscopy: intraductal tubular neoplasm.

Infiltrated or ulcerated strictures
Papillary mucosal projections
Villous mucosal projections

COMPARATIVE STUDIES

No randomized studies have been performed to compare peroral CP with ERCP or percutaneous cholangioscopy. These avenues of cholangiopancreatopic approach are based on multiple factors: primarily the location of pathologic conditions, patient factors, and availability of resources (ie, cholangioscopes, availability of collaborative interventional gastroenterologists, and radiologists). In general, most biliary stone disease will be tackled with routine ERCP extraction methods. When this approach fails, stone clearance with ESWL and ERCP revealed 79% stone clearance compared with an equally effective clearance rate of 74% with peroral cholangioscopy with EHL,

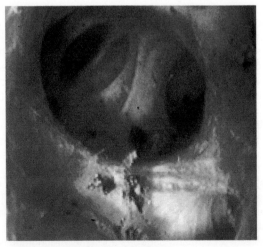

Fig. 10. Percutaneous tract into the intrahepatic ducts.

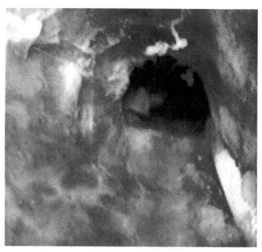

Fig. 11. Percutaneous tract with wire leading into the liver.

in a nonrandomized group of 125 patients with CBD stones with previous attempts at conventional endoscopic treatment.[48] However, the ESWL group had the disadvantages of having 2 treatments compared with one treatment with EHL, and needing ERCP performed after each treatment to extract stone fragments.[48]

A retrospective evaluation of 59 patients with hepatolithiasis compared percutaneous cholangioscopy with EHL with selective hepatic resection.[49] Resection was considered in settings of unilateral stones, an atrophic lobe or segment, or suspicion of cholangiocarcinoma, whereas EHL was considered for right-sided, bilateral, or recurrent stone disease and if resection was refused. Stone clearance was high, at 96% in both groups, with a comparable 30-day complication rate and 5-year survival. However, there were 3 deaths (12%) in the resection group, 2 of which were related to

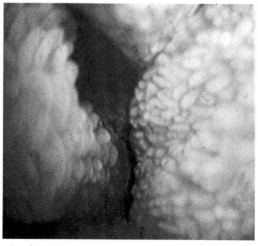

Fig. 12. Papillary fronds of IPMN as seen on choledochoscopy.

delayed liver failure. In the EHL group there was 1 death (4%) from massive hemobilia and a statistically significantly higher recurrence rate of hepatolithiasis, 32% versus 6%, in the operative group.

UTILITY AND LIMITATIONS

Several obstacles prohibit CP from widespread use. Need for additional training and expertise, increased procedure time, and fragile scope design are the most common limiting factors. Because the cholangiopancreatoscope has a 10F diameter, this limits its capability to cannulate an intact sphincter, and to traverse narrow ducts and tight strictures. Complete ductal inspection may be achieved with a 2- or 4-way deflection tip with the application of torque on the duodenoscope. However, using the accessory channel is challenging and sometimes inhibited by angulations in the scope, narrow duct diameter, and strictures. If the ducts are significantly dilated, complete visualization is limited by its narrow field of view. During visual inspection the operator must take note of any prior stent placement, ERCP-guided biopsies, or postdilation changes, as this can change the topographic appearance and limit an accurate diagnosis.

SUMMARY

CP is a well-established modality for the direct visualization of intrahepatic biliary, extrahepatic biliary, and pancreatic ductal systems. The utility of CP in the treatment of difficult biliary stones has become paramount when standard ERCP is ineffective. Intraductal tissue sampling in the hands of experienced endoscopists increases diagnostic yields when evaluating suspicious strictures and mapping for cholangiocarcinoma. The peroral route of cholangioscopy has lower morbidity rates; therefore the percutaneous route should be reserved for cases inaccessible from the peroral approach, needing intraductal lithotripsy and tissue sampling.

REFERENCES

1. McIver MA. An instrument for visualizing the interior of the common duct at operation. Surgery 1941;9:112–4.
2. Bower BL, Picus D, Hicks ME, et al. Choledochoscopic stone removal through a T-tube tract: experience in 75 consecutive patients. J Vasc Interv Radiol 1990;1:107–12.
3. Palayew MJ, Stein L. Postoperative biopsy of the common bile duct via the T-tube tract. AJR Am J Roentgenol 1978;130:287–9.
4. Ponchon T, Genin G, Mitchell R, et al. Methods, indications, and results of percutaneous choledochoscopy: a series of 161 procedures. Ann Surg 1996;223:26–36.
5. Vennes JA, Silvis SE. Endoscopic visualization of bile and pancreatic ducts. Gastrointest Endosc 1972;18:149–52.
6. Nakajima M, Akasaka Y, Yamaguchi K, et al. Direct endoscopic visualization of the bile and pancreatic duct systems by peroral cholangiopancreatoscopy (PCPS). Gastrointest Endsoc 1978;24:141–5.
7. Shah RJ, Langer DA, Antillon MR, et al. Cholangioscopy and cholangioscopic forceps biopsy in patients with indeterminate pancreaticobiliary pathology. Clin Gastroenterol Hepatol 2006;4:219–25.

8. Piraka C, Shah RJ, Awadallah, et al. Transpapillary cholangioscopy directed lithotripsy in patients with difficult bile duct stones. Clin Gastroenterol Hepatol 2007; 5:1333–8.

9. Arya N, Nelles SE, Haber GB, et al. Electrohydraulic lithotripsy in 111 patients: a safe and effective therapy for difficult bile duct stones. Am J Gastroenterol 2004;99:2330–4.

10. Soda K, Shitou K, Yoshida Y, et al. Peroral cholangioscopy using a new fine-caliber flexible scope for detailed examination without papillotomy. Gastrointest Endsoc 1996;43:233–8.

11. ASGE Technology Status Evaluation. Cholangiopancreatoscopy. Gastrointest Endosc 2008;68(3):411–21.

12. Larghi A, Waxman I. Endoscopic direct cholangioscopy by using an ultra-slim upper endoscope: a feasibility study. Gastrointest Endosc 2006;63:853–7.

13. Urakami Y, Seifert E, Butke H. Peroral direct cholangioscopy using routine straight-view endoscope: first report. Endoscopy 1977;9:27–30.

14. Somogyi L, Dimashkieh H, Weber FL, et al. Biliary intraductal papillary mucinous tumor: diagnosis and localization by endoscopic retrograde cholangioscopy. Gastrointest Endosc 2003;57:620–2.

15. Lew RJ, Kochman ML. Video cholangioscopy with a new choledochoscope: a case report. Gastrointest Endosc 2003;57:804–7.

16. Kodama T, Tatsumi Y, Sato H, et al. Initial experience with a new peroral electronic pancreatoscope with an accessory channel. Gastrointest Endosc 2004;59: 895–900.

17. Itoi T, Sofuni A, Itokawa F, et al. Peroral cholangioscopic diagnosis of biliary-tract diseases by using narrow-band imaging (with videos). Gastrointest Endosc 2007; 66:730–6.

18. Seibel EJ, Brentnall TA, Dominitz JA. New endoscopic and cytologic tools for cancer surveillance in the digestive tract. Gastrointest Endosc Clin N Am 2009; 19(2):299–307.

19. Seibel EJ, Brown CM, Dominitz JA, et al. Scanning single fiber endoscopy: a new platform technology for integrated laser imaging, diagnosis, and future therapies. Gastrointest Endosc Clin N Am 2008;18:467–78.

20. Farrell JJ, Bounds BC, Al-Shalabi S, et al. Single-operator duodenoscope-assisted cholangioscopy is an effective alternative in the management of choledocholithiasis not removed by conventional methods, including mechanical lithotripsy. Endoscopy 2005;37:542–7.

21. Siddique I, Galati J, Ankoma-Sey V, et al. The role of choledochoscopy in the diagnosis and management of biliary tract disease. Gastrointest Endosc 1999; 50:67–73.

22. Seo DW, Lee SK, Yoo KS, et al. Cholangioscopic findings in bile duct tumors. Gastrointest Endosc 2000;52:630–4.

23. Bonnel DH, Liguory CE, Cornud FE, et al. Common bile duct and intrahepatic stones: results of transhepatic, electrohydraulic lithotripsy in 50 patients. Radiology 1991;180:345–8.

24. Lee SK, Seo DW, Myung SJ. Percutaneous transhepatic cholangioscopic treatment for hepatolithiasis: an evaluation of long-term results and risk factors for recurrence. Gastrointest Endosc 2001;53:318–23.

25. Andrea W, Gouchen J. Complications of percutaneous transhepatic biliary drainage in patients with dilated and nondilated intrahepatic bile ducts. Eur J Radiol 2008;62:1.

26. Hwang MH, Tsai CC, Mo LR, et al. Percutaneous choledochoscopic biliary tract stone removal: experience in 645 consecutive patients. Eur J Radiol 1993;17: 184–90.

27. Tamada K, Kurihara K, Tomiyama T, et al. How many biopsies should be performed during percutaneous transhepatic cholangioscopy to diagnose biliary tract cancer? Gastrointest Endosc 1999;50:653–8.

28. Tamada K, Tomiyama T, Ohashi A. Access for percutaneous cholangioscopy in patients with nondilated bile ducts using nasobiliary catheter cholangiography and oblique fluoroscopy. Gastrointest Endosc 2000;52:765–70.

29. Sievert CE, Silvis SE. Evaluation of electrohydraulic lithotripsy as a means of gallstone fragmentation in a canine model. Gastrointest Endosc 1987;33:233–5.

30. Harrison J, Morris DL, Haynes J. Electrohydraulic lithotripsy of gallstones—in vitro and animal studies. Gut 1987;28:267–71.

31. Oi I, Kobayashi S, Kondo T. Endoscopic pancreatocholangiography. Endoscopy 1970;2:103–6 and [Kawai K, Akasaka Y. Endoscopic sphincterotomy of the ampulla of Vater. Gastrointest Endosc 1974;20:148–51.]

32. Kawai K, Nakajima M, Akasaka Y, et al. A new endoscopic method: the peroral choledocho-pancreatoscopy. [author's translation]. Leber Magen Darm 1976;6:121–4.

33. Bar-Meir S, Rotmensch S. A comparison between peroral choledochoscopy and endoscopic retrograde cholangiopancreatography. Gastrointestinal Endosc 1987;33:13–4.

34. Nora PF, Berci G, Dorazio RA, et al. Operative choledochoscopy: results of a prospective study in several institutions. Am J Surg 1977;133:105–10.

35. Giurgiu DI, Margulies DR, Carroll BJ, et al. Laparoscopic common bile duct exploration: long-term outcome. Arch Surg 1999;134:839–43.

36. Arregui ME, Davis CJ, Arkush AM, et al. Laparoscopic cholecystectomy combined with endoscopic sphincterotomy and stone extraction or laparoscopic choledochoscopy and electrohydraulic lithotripsy for management of cholelithiasis with choledocholithiasis. Surg Endosc 1992;6:10–5.

37. Lau WY, Chu KW, Yuen WK, et al. Operative choledochoscopy in patients with acute cholangitis: a prospective, randomized study. Br J Surg 1991;78:1226–9.

38. Rios GA, Adams DB. Does intraoperative electrohydraulic lithotripsy improve outcome in the surgical management of chronic pancreatitis? Am Surg 2001; 67:533–7.

39. Kaneko T, Nakao A, Nomoto S, et al. Intraoperative pancreatoscopy with the ultrathin pancreatoscope for mucin-producing tumors of the pancreas. Arch Surg 1998;133:263–7.

40. Okugawa T, Tsuyuguchi T, Sudhamshu KC, et al. Peroral cholangioscopic treatment of hepatolithiasis: long-term results. Gastrointest Endsoc 2002;56:366–71.

41. Awadallah NS, Chen YK, Piraka C, et al. Is there a role for cholangioscopy in patients with primary sclerosing cholangitis? Am J Gastroenterol 2006;101:284–91.

42. Huang MH, Chen CH, Yang JC, et al. Long-term outcome of percutaneous transhepatic cholangioscopic lithotomy for hepatolithiasis. Am J Gastroenterol 2003; 98:2655–62.

43. Kim HJ, Kim MH, Lee SK, et al. Tumor vessel: a valuable cholangioscopic clue of malignant biliary stricture. Gastrointest Endosc 2000;52:635–8.

44. Craigie JE, Adams DB, Byme TK, et al. Endoscopic electrohydraulic lithotripsy in the management of pancreatobiliary lithiasis. Surg Endosc 1998;12:405–8.

45. Howell DA, Dy RM, Hanson BL, et al. Endoscopic treatment of pancreatic duct stones using a 10F pancreatoscope and electrohydraulic lithotripsy. Gastrointest Endosc 1999;50:829–33.

46. Yamao K, Ohashi K, Nakamura T, et al. Efficacy of peroral pancreatoscopy in the diagnosis of pancreatic diseases. Gastrointest Endosc 2003;57:205–9.
47. Kodama T, Imamura Y, Sato H, et al. Feasibility study using a new small electronic pancreatoscope: description of findings in chronic pancreatitis. Endoscopy 2003;35:305–10.
48. Adamek HE, Maier M, Jakobs R, et al. Management of retained bile duct stones: a prospective open trial comparing extracorporeal and intracorporeal lithotripsy. Gastrointest Endosc 1996;44:40–7.
49. Otani K, Shimizu S, Chijiiwa K, et al. Comparison of treatments for hepatolithiasis: hepatic resection versus cholangioscopic lithotomy. J Am Coll Surg 1999;189: 177–82.

New Kid on the Block: Development of a Partially Disposable System for Cholangioscopy

Krishnavel V. Chathadi, MD[a,b], Yang K. Chen, MD[a,c,d],*

KEYWORDS

- Cholangioscopy • SpyGlass • ERCP • EHL • Directed biopsy
- Biliary stricture • Biliary stone

HISTORY AND EVOLUTION OF CHOLANGIOSCOPY

Cholangioscopy allows for direct visualization of the bile duct using a miniature endoscope. It was first performed more than 60 years ago during surgical open bile-duct exploration for intraoperative localization of stones.[1] Early diagnostic and therapeutic cholangioscopy was performed through either a surgically created or percutaneous biliary access.[2–7] Duodenoscope-assisted retrograde cholangioscopy with the mother-daughter system, as we know it, was first performed in the early eighties.[8] Early retrograde cholangioscopy, however, used a specially designed large-channel duodenoscope to accommodate the cholangioscope.[9] Improvements in optics, scope diameter, and tip deflection have since enabled the development of cholangioscopes that are capable of being passed through the working channel of a standard therapeutic duodenoscope.[10]

Several diagnostic and therapeutic clinical applications have driven the evolution of cholangioscopy. Diagnostic indications include evaluation of equivocal fluoroscopy findings, characterization and directed tissue sampling of strictures (including

[a] Division of Gastroenterology and Hepatology, Department of Medicine, University of Colorado Denver, MS 735, 1653 Aurora Court, Room AIP 2.031, Aurora, CO 80045, USA
[b] Division of Gastroenterology, Department of Medicine, Denver Health Medical Center, 777 Bannock Street, Mail Code 4000, Denver, CO 80204, USA
[c] Department of Medicine, University of Colorado Hospital, 12605 E. 16th Avenue, Aurora, CO 80045, USA
[d] University of Colorado Denver, MS 735, 1635 Aurora Court, Room AIP 2.031, Aurora, CO 80045, USA
* Corresponding author. University of Colorado Denver, MS 735, 1635 Aurora Court, Room AIP 2.031, Aurora, CO 80045.
E-mail address: yang.chen@ucdenver.edu (Y.K. Chen).

Gastrointest Endoscopy Clin N Am 19 (2009) 545–555
doi:10.1016/j.giec.2009.06.001
1052-5157/09/$ – see front matter © 2009 Elsevier Inc. All rights reserved.

determination of morphologic features and extent of cholangiocarcinoma), and detection of occult stones.[9] Therapeutic indications include treatment of difficult biliary stones, palliative therapy of biliary malignancies,[11] and facilitation of selective guidewire access to the gallbladder or intrahepatic ducts.

LIMITATIONS OF CHOLANGIOSCOPY BEFORE SPYGLASS

Despite the availability of cholangioscopes, direct visualization of the pancreatobiliary system for diagnosis and therapy has not been widely applied in clinical practice thus far because of technical and technological limitations. These limitations, including suboptimal functionality and lack of user-friendliness of the available systems, have confined its use to select academic centers. For example, these cholangioscopy systems required 2 trained operators; 1 physician to handle the "mother" duodenoscope, the other to maneuver the "daughter" cholangioscope. This procedure took extra time, patience, and coordination between 2 physicians. In addition, these traditional cholangioscopes were capable of only 2-way steering, which limited the field of view. A single small working channel was also taxed by having to deliver irrigation as well as access guidewire and any other desired accessory, such as a probe for laser or electrohydraulic lithotripsy (EHL) or biopsy forceps for tissue sampling. These cholangioscopes also had thin steering cables and a fragile fiberoptic bundle, and they were susceptible to rupture of the scope's outer sheath, particularly at the bending section. Damage to the scope was common after just a few uses. Repairs were costly and could be as high as 35% to 50% of the original cost of the scope. Tissue acquisition was tedious because of lack of high-quality forceps that could reliably obtain adequate tissue samples. Lack of 4-way tip deflection made it more difficult to pinpoint a lesion of interest for tissue sampling or treatment. Sharp angulations often prevented access into intrahepatic ducts, the cystic duct, and the pancreatic duct. Maintaining a sufficient volume of fluid in the duct, while using an EHL probe, all through a Luer-lock port on the single working channel was also challenging. These procedures were successful only in the best of hands.

SPYGLASS DIRECT VISUALIZATION SYSTEM FEATURES AND DESCRIPTION

Although the clinical value of optically guided biliary diagnosis and intervention was obvious, failure to overcome these technical handicaps limited advancement in this field. The SpyGlass Direct Visualization System (SDVS) was designed to address many of these issues by being the first single-use direct visualization system requiring only 1 physician operator, featuring dedicated irrigation and therapeutic channels, and providing 4-way steerability in a sturdy 4-lumen single-use catheter.

The SDVS is an integrated product platform that combines capital components and consumable devices to provide an endoluminal view for directing therapeutic devices within the biliary duct system.[12] The capital components are housed in a tower comprising a cart, irrigation pump, camera, light source, and monitor. A light cable and camera cable plug into the front of the respective units and then attach to a focusing ocular held by a flexible 3-joint arm assembly (**Fig. 1**). The SpyGlass Direct Visualization Probe (SDVP) is a reusable fiberoptic probe with average use of about 8 to 10 times. The SpyGlass Probe (SP) contains a 6000-pixel image bundle surrounded by approximately 225 light transmission fibers.[13] The image bundle and light fibers are covered by an outer sheath that is engineered for flexibility and reduction of friction when it is pushed through the optic channel of the SpyScope Access and Delivery Catheter (SADC). This design bonds these fibers as 1 bundle, reducing breakage of individual fibers. One advantage with this design is that one will not see lost pixels

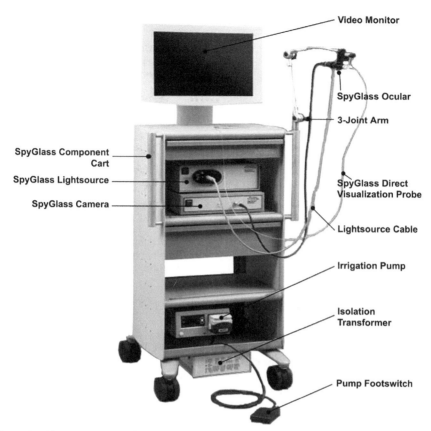

Fig. 1. SpyGlass Direct Visualization capital components. (*Courtesy of* Boston Scientific, Natick, MA, USA; with permission.)

or little black dots on the screen. A lens connected to the image bundle at the distal tip captures images across a 70° field of view. At its proximal end in the SpyGlass Ocular (SO), the probe connects to the light and ocular cables that provide the mechanical and optical interface between the probe and the video camera head and light source. The SDVP enters the biliary anatomy through the SADC that is attached to a duodeno-scope. The SP may be reused after high-level disinfection. The single-use SADC (10F in diameter and 230 cm in length) is designed to provide a pathway into the biliary anatomy for diagnostic and therapeutic devices (**Fig. 2**).[14] It contains a flexible delivery catheter with a handle housing 2 articulating knobs to provide 4-way tip deflection. The catheter has 4 open lumens: one 1-mm optic channel through which the SP is passed, one 1.2-mm working device channel that delivers devices or guidewire, and 2 irrigation channels that merge in the handle assembly (**Fig. 3**). The SpyScope Cath-eter (SC) attaches to a standard duodenoscope with a 4.2-mm working channel, which allows a single physician to manage both scopes. The 4-way tip deflection at the tip of the SC has a short turning radius, engineered to enhance directional control and permit more precise navigation within the biliary anatomy. The original SpyScope (version 1.0) had limited tip flexibility, and this reduced its maneuverability in the duct. Soon after the launch of the SpyGlass System, an improved version (version 1.5) was released with greater tip articulation range. The SpyBite Biopsy Forceps (SBF) are

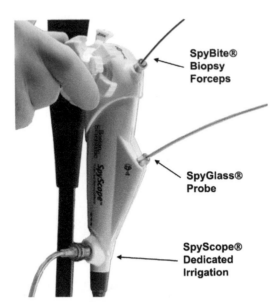

Fig. 2. SpyScope Access and Delivery Catheter. (*Courtesy of* Boston Scientific, Natick, MA, USA; with permission.)

miniature forceps that are introduced through the 1.2-mm working channel of the Spy-Scope (see **Fig. 3**). The jaw outer diameter is 1 mm, with 4.1 mm/55° jaw opening. These forceps obtain adequate tissue for diagnoses; however, the volume of the tissue is similar to cardiac biopsies. Pathology laboratories in most hospitals have a separate handling procedure for these very small tissue samples.

TECHNIQUE FOR USING THE SPYGLASS SYSTEM IN CHOLANGIOSCOPY

The cholangioscopy procedure using the SpyGlass System is performed by a single operator, by strapping the SADC to the handle of the duodenoscope just below the operating channel (see **Fig. 2**). In this configuration, the endoscopist controls the tip deflection wheels of both the duodenoscope and the SC visualization system with

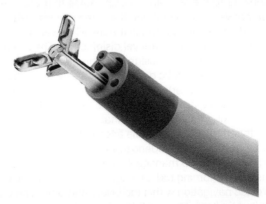

Fig. 3. SpyBite Biopsy Forceps and Spyglass Direct Visualization Probe exiting through distal end of SpyScope Access and Delivery Catheter. (*Courtesy of* Boston Scientific, Natick, MA, USA; with permission.)

the right hand. The physician's left hand holds the duodenoscope to stabilize both systems and to torque the duodenoscope as needed. Preloading the SDVP into the optic channel of the SC is recommended, with the tip of the probe positioned approximately midway into the bending section of the SC. Then the catheter and optical probe are introduced as a unit through the duodenoscope (**Fig. 4**), typically by backloading it over a 0.035-in guide wire already positioned in the duct of interest. A biliary sphincterotomy is usually required to facilitate passage into the duct; elevator use should be avoided as this may cause damage to the catheter/probe. The SC and SP are maneuvered up to the area of interest within the duct for direct visualization (**Fig. 5**). Once inside the duct, the guidewire can be removed and the probe advanced to a position just beyond the tip of the catheter. Small controlled movements of the knobs will direct the tip of the SpyScope. There is a friction brake that locks to the knobs and helps to maintain the desired catheter tip position. Selected ducts and branches of interest can be systematically examined during repeated advancement and withdrawal of the system. Once inside the duct, intermittent water irrigation will help to clear the field by flushing out tissue debris, blood, or stone fragments. An irrigation pump equipped with a pump foot switch is connected to the SC for this purpose (see **Figs. 1** and **2**). A syringe could also be attached to the 1.2-mm operating channel to provide suction or additional manual irrigation. To aid in duct clearance while irrigating, the operator can simultaneously apply intermittent gentle suction with the duodenoscope to draw the fluid from the biliary system. This maneuver provides a satisfactory lavage effect and is critical to optimizing the image (**Fig. 6**). Because the dedicated irrigation channels of the SC provide a maximum flow rate that is severalfold higher than what is possible with conventional single-channel cholangioscopes,[15] vigorous irrigation across an obstructed duct should be avoided to minimize the risk of cholangitis. If indicated, the SBF can be introduced through the 1.2-mm operating channel to procure biopsies under direct visual guidance.

A small 3F EHL probe is passed through the working channel of the SC to treat difficult stones. Under direct visualization, the lithotripsy probe is advanced until it comes into contact with the target stone. Water is infused through the dedicated irrigation channels to provide a fluid environment. EHL is applied until the stones are broken into multiple small fragments. Then standard stone extraction devices and techniques are used to clear the ducts of remaining stone fragments. A cholangiogram is taken to confirm that the bile duct is clear. Recently, an improved version of the biliary EHL probe (Northgate Technologies Inc, Elgin, IL) was released for clinical use; the new

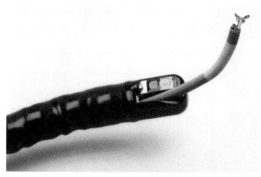

Fig. 4. SpyScope Access and Delivery Catheter exiting through distal end of duodenoscope. (*Courtesy of* Boston Scientific, Natick, MA, USA; with permission.)

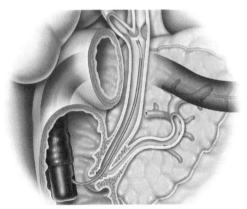

Fig. 5. Schematic of SpyGlass evaluation of a hilar stricture. (*Courtesy of* Boston Scientific, Natick, MA, USA; with permission.)

probe provides a longer working length (375 cm vs 250 cm), a beveled tip for easier passage through the bending section of the SpyScope, and a stiffer probe with reinforcement of the proximal shaft to minimize kinking. Holmium laser lithotripsy can also be performed for the same indications.

PRECLINICAL STUDY

The initial studies with SpyGlass helped to define the design and later verified safety and efficacy. During preclinical characterization, the SDVS was evaluated by bench simulation and porcine model experiments.[15] The capabilities of the SpyGlass System for direct access, visualization, and biopsy in all quadrants were compared with those of a control fiberoptic choledochoscope with 2-way deflection (CHF-BP30; Olympus America Inc, Center Valley, PA) using an innovative bench simulator, with the cholangioscopes inserted through a duodenoscope in a standard endoscopic retrograde cholangiopancreatography (ERCP) position. The study demonstrated that 4-way

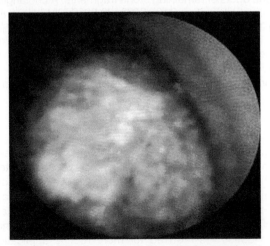

Fig. 6. Stone in the common bile duct as seen through the SpyGlass System. (*Courtesy of* Boston Scientific, Natick, MA, USA; with permission.)

deflection can allow access to all 4 quadrants of the bile duct, with or without forceps loaded, to visualize and obtain biopsies from simulated targets. As could have been predicted, the control system endowed with only 2-way deflection permitted access to only approximately half the quadrants and biopsy targets and its success rate for simulated biopsy was only approximately a third of the success rate of the SpyGlass system. Flow rates of irrigation fluid through the SpyScope were compared with those through 2 control cholangioscopes (CHF-BP30, Olympus; and FCP-9P, Pentax Medical Co, Montvale, NJ). Laboratory measurements in this study indicated that, with biopsy forceps loaded, the dedicated irrigation channels of the SpyGlass System can produce flow rates 4 to 5 times those attained through the working channel of conventional systems. In addition, a standardized test target (1951 USAF Glass Slide Resolution Targets; Edmund Optics Inc, Barrington, NJ) was visually evaluated at a distance of 5 mm to compare the optical resolution of the SpyGlass Optical Probe (SOP) and the Olympus cholangioscope. The measured optical resolution of the SOP was twice that of the conventional fiberoptic cholangioscope. With regard to high-level disinfection of the reusable optical probe, a 6-log or greater reduction in the number of test organisms after high-level disinfection of SOPs was attained in this study. These results were obtained after 20 reprocessing cycles, thus indicating the durability of the probes. Furthermore, surface integrity and optical resolution were maintained during reprocessing, affirming the suitability of the SOPs for repeated use. In the porcine model, SpyGlass-directed biopsies were performed, 14 above and 20 below the hepatic bifurcation. Adequate gross specimen was secured in 91% of biopsies. The quality of 90% of the specimens was also rated adequate to excellent for histologic examination.

FIRST HUMAN USE

Results from the first human use series provided the first clinical evidence that the SpyGlass System is safe and technically feasible.[16] Consecutive SpyGlass examinations were performed in 35 patients undergoing ERCP at 2 centers. Indications for peroral cholangioscopy included indeterminate strictures, indeterminate filling defects, EHL stone therapy, evaluation of cystic lesions, and gallbladder stenting. The rate of procedural success was 91%; access to some areas of interest was precluded by small intrahepatic duct size in 2 patients, and visualization of a short presphincteric stricture was suboptimal in another patient. SpyBite biopsies were performed in 20 patients, and 95% were adequate for histologic diagnosis. SpyGlass-directed EHL achieved stone clearance in all 5 patients who had previously failed conventional ERCP stone removal. The preliminary sensitivity and specificity of SpyGlass-directed biopsy to diagnose malignancy (based on 6 months of follow-up) were 71% and 100%, respectively. Procedure-related complications occurred in 2 patients and resolved uneventfully.

SPYGLASS REGISTRY

The largest case series on cholangioscopy has been completed. A 15-center international registry has documented the performance and utility of peroral cholangioscopy using the SpyGlass System in 297 patients requiring the procedure for stone therapy or investigation of suspected biliary pathology.[17–19] Twelve-month follow-up data will be completed on the registry patients by April 2009. Interim results from this registry (N = 296) were presented at Digestive Disease Week in San Diego on May 20, 2008. The primary selection criterion of the study was indication for ERCP/cholangioscopy with or without biopsy. The primary endpoint was procedural success—defined as the ability to visualize stricture and obtain biopsy adequate for histologic examination for stricture and suspected malignancy cases or the ability to visualize stones and successfully initiate stone fragmentation and removal for stone cases. Secondary endpoints included the effect of cholangioscopy on diagnosis and patient management and the sensitivity and specificity of biopsy. The mean age was 63 years, and 51% were women. The SpyGlass System was used only for visualization in 56 cases, 137 had a SpyBite Biopsy attempt, 98 had stone treatment, and 5 had failed access.

The primary indications for SpyGlass were indeterminate strictures (35.9%), stone management only (31.9%), exclusion of malignancy in primary sclerosing cholangitis (10.5%), indeterminate filling defect (6.4%), other nondiagnostic findings (5.4%), and unclassified (9.8%). Results of the procedural success were 88% overall: 92% in the stones with EHL/laser lithotripsy group (mean stone size 19 mm); 93% in the stones with conventional (mechanical) lithotripsy/extraction group (mean stone size 10 mm); 96% in the stricture/suspected malignancy without biopsy group (visual assessment only); and 86% in the stricture/suspected malignancy with biopsy group. Access to target site was unsuccessful in 5 cases, and data was missing in 8. Each case was performed by a single operator. Visual diagnosis was discordant from ERCP diagnosis in 19%. SpyGlass System visual impression versus malignancy at complete follow-up (12 mo) was available on 43 patients with an accuracy of 86% (37/43) and sensitivity of 90% (35/39). Of the 137 patients who had biopsies using the SBF (mean number of biopsies 4.3), 124 had complete baseline data, including histology. Patients with a benign biopsy were followed up until a definitive malignant diagnosis was made or 12 months had passed. In this subgroup of biopsy of indeterminate biliary strictures, procedural success was 86% (based on intention to treat analysis). In the subgroup of 98 patients who had peroral cholangioscopic-guided stone therapy, per protocol, each patient had ERCP immediately followed by cholangioscopy-guided stone therapy using the SDVS. In 29% of cases, stones were missed during the ERCP immediately preceding cholangioscopy. Overall, only 23 serious adverse events were reported in 296 patients, with cholangitis being the most frequent complication (2.4%).

Hence, interim results from this registry demonstrated that SpyGlass cholangioscopy was safe, that it had a high rate of procedural success, and that direct visualization improved the accuracy of cholangiographic findings when used in conjunction with ERCP. Direct visualization had a good diagnostic predictive value in patients with biliary obstructive symptoms of indeterminate origin. It was also noted that the rate of missed stones by ERCP might be higher than previously reported. Cholangioscopy is useful for directing lithotripsy of difficult bile duct stones and is facilitated by the availability of dedicated irrigation capabilities. Cholangioscopy-guided bile duct biopsies provided specimens adequate for histologic examination in most cases (86%). The final results of cholangioscopy-guided biopsy, using the SBF for diagnosing indeterminate biliary strictures, are awaiting completion of 12-month follow-up.

OTHER APPLICATIONS OF SPYGLASS

SpyGlass cholangioscopy has been reported to be superior to cholangiography in demonstrating anastomotic patency in liver transplant recipients.[20] SpyGlass was used successfully to enter the cystic duct for guidewire placement and gallbladder stenting in a patient with pretransplant cirrhosis and symptomatic cholelithiasis who had previously failed multiple attempts to cannulate the cystic duct for gallbladder stenting at ERCP.[16] Similarly, the system was used to place a guidewire across a tight anastomotic stricture after earlier failed attempts to cannulate the stricture at ERCP.[21] SpyGlass-directed biopsy was reported to obtain a diagnosis of biliary sarcoidosis in a patient with Klatskin-like hilar obstruction.[22] Peroral cholangioscopy using the SDVS has also been used to detect a T-tube remnant in the cystic duct that had failed earlier detection by computed tomography, magnetic resonance cholangiopancreatography, and ERCP, facilitating subsequent removal by balloon sweep in a patient with recurrent pancreatitis.[23] The SOP has been used in conjunction with a endoscopic ultrasound–guided fine needle aspiration (EUS-FNA) needle in a "needlescopy" approach within pancreatic and gastric cysts.[24]

FUTURE

The SDVS offers several unique features, including a single-operator design, 4-way tip deflection, and dedicated irrigation channels, which conventional cholangioscopes do not have. However, there are opportunities to improve this system. The most obvious need is for improved image quality. The fiberoptic images of the current SDVS are inferior in quality to digital images routinely acquired in the gastrointestinal tract with standard video endoscopes.[25] Although fiberoptic images are acceptable for target recognition and delivery of therapy, differentiating benign from malignant biliary lesions will likely require higher-quality digital images in many instances. With recent developments in charge-coupled device chip technology, mass-producing single-use SpyGlass digital cholangioscopes is now feasible. Because the SpyScope and the SOP are not fused, the probe may retract slightly during SpyScope turning, necessitating readjustment during the procedure. Conversion to digital technology will overcome the procedural challenges of using such a modular system and dispense with the need to reprocess a fragile optical probe. To ensure a crisp image, the SO has to be manually refocused during equipment setup. Manual adjustment of light intensity is also required because the current light source lacks an automated gain and light function for changing illumination circumstances. As is true of conventional cholangioscopes, the SpyScope has no suction capability, although manual suction can be achieved by attaching a syringe to the operating channel and applying negative pressure.

The future of biliary endoscopy will undoubtedly rely on direct visualization technologies to deliver novel diagnostic modalities and therapies. Some day we will look back on fluoroscopy as an antiquated visualization method (as we do today with barium enemas) and realize that through miniature imaging technology, so much more is possible in the pancreatobiliary space. We are a little closer to realizing that dream, thanks to this new kid on the block.

ACKNOWLEDGMENTS

The authors would like to thank Boston Scientific Corporation for providing the figures used in this article.

REFERENCES

1. McIver MA. An instrument for visualizing the interior of the common duct at operation. Surgery 1941;9:112–4.
2. Stellato T. Flexible endoscope as an adjunct to laparoscopic surgery. Surg Clin North Am 1996;76:595–602.

3. Stage JG, Moesgard F, Gronvall S, et al. Percutaneous transhepatic cholelitho-tripsy for difficult common bile duct stones. Endoscopy 1998;30:289–92.
4. Ponchon T, Genin G, Mitchell R, et al. Methods, indications, and results of percu-taneous choledochoscopy: a series of 161 procedures. Ann Surg 1996;223: 26–36.
5. Picus D. Percutaneous biliary endoscopy. J Vasc Interv Radiol 1995;6:303–10.
6. Khoo DE, Walsh CJ, Cox MR, et al. Laparoscopic common bile duct exploration: evolution of a new technique. Br J Surg 1996;83:341–6.
7. Ferguson C. Laparoscopic common bile duct exploration: practical application. Arch Surg 1998;133:448–51.
8. Nelson DB, Bosco JJ, Curtis WD, et al. Duodenoscope-assisted cholangiopan-creatoscopy. Gastrointest Endosc 1999;50(6):943–5.
9. Shah RJ, Adler DG, Conway JD, et al. Cholangiopancreatoscopy. Technology status evaluation report. Gastrointest Endosc 2008;68(3):411–21.
10. Soda K, Shitou K, Yoshida Y, et al. Peroral cholangioscopy using a new fine-caliber flexible scope for detailed examination without papillotomy. Gastrointest Endosc 1996;43:233–8.
11. Brauer BC, Fukami N, Chen YK. Direct cholangioscopy with narrow band imaging, chromoendoscopy, and argon plasma coagulation of intraductal papil-lary mucinous neoplasm of the bile duct (with videos). Gastrointest Endosc 2008; 67(3):574–6.
12. SpyGlass Direct Visualization System [brochure]. Natick (MA): Boston Scientific Corporation; 2007. SME11280 500 5/07.
13. SpyGlass Direct Visualization Probe [brochure]. Natick (MA): Boston Scientific Corporation; 2007. DVG1820 500 5/07.
14. SpyScope Access and Delivery Catheter [brochure]. Natick (MA): Boston Scien-tific Corporation; 2007. DVG1830 500 5/07.
15. Chen YK. Preclinical characterization of the SpyGlass peroral cholangiopancrea-toscopy system for direct access, visualization and biopsy. Gastrointest Endosc 2007;65:301–11.
16. Chen YK, Pleskow DK. SpyGlass singe-operator peroral cholangiopancreato-scopy system for the diagnosis and therapy for bile-duct disorders: a clinical feasibility study. (with video). Gastrointest Endosc 2007;65:832–41.
17. Chen YK, Parsi MA, Neuhas H, et al. Peroral Cholangioscopy (PO) using a dispos-able steerable single operator catheter for biliary stone therapy and assessment of indeterminate strictures – a multi-center experience using spyglass [abstract]. Gastrointest Endosc 2008;67(5):103.
18. Pleskow D, Parsi M, Binmoeller K, et al. Biopsy of indeterminate biliary strictures – does direct visualization help? A multicenter experience [abstract]. Gastrointest Endosc 2008;67(5):103.
19. Parsi M, Neuhas H, Chen YK, et al. Peroral cholangioscopy guided stone therapy- report of an international multicenter registry [abstract]. Gastrointest Endosc 2008;67(5):102.
20. Kim JJ, Yee S, Yang RD. The utility of spyglass choledochoscopy for evaluation of suspected post-liver transplant strictures [abstract 170]. Am J Gastroenterol 2008;103:S66.
21. Wright H, Sharad S, Jabbour N, et al. Management of biliary stricture by the Spyglass direct visualization system in a liver transplant recipient: an innovative approach. Gastrointest Endosc 2008;67(3):1201–3.
22. Petersen JM. Klatskin-like biliary sarcoidosis – a spyglass diagnosis [abstract 599]. Am J Gastroenterol 2008;103:S232.

23. Parsi M, Sanaka MR, Dumont JA. Iatrogenic recurrent pancreatitis. Pancreatology 2007;7(5-6):539.
24. Antillon M, Tiwari P, Marshall J, et al. Taking SpyGlass outside the GI tract lumen in conjunction with EUS to assist in the diagnosis of a pancreatic cystic lesion. (with video). Gastrointest Endosc 2009;69(3):591–3.
25. Draganov P. The spyglass direct visualization system for cholangioscopy. Gastroenterology & Hepatology 2008;4(7):469–70.

Diagnostic Value of Image-Enhanced Video Cholangiopancreatoscopy

Takao Itoi, MD[a],*, Horst Neuhaus, MD[b], Yang K. Chen, MD[c]

KEYWORDS

- Cholangioscopy • Pancreatoscopy • Narrow-band imaging
- Chromoendoscopy • Image-enhanced endoscopy

Peroral cholangiopancreatoscopy (PCPS)[1–7] and percutaneous transhepatic cholangioscopy (PTCS)[8–13] have been developed over the past three decades to enable direct endoscopic observation of bile duct lesions or pancreatic duct lesions that are difficult to evaluate by cholangiopancreatography, and to guide tissue sampling. However, both PCPS and PTCS have also been used for therapeutic indications. Previously, the image resolution was limited using the fiberoptic systems. To overcome this problem, a video cholangiopancreatoscope was developed approximately one decade ago.[14–17] Video cholangiopancreatoscopes provides better quality digital images and offers enhanced mucosal detail (**Table 1**). To date, two video PCPSs (CHF-B260 and CHF-BP260, with outer diameters of 3.4 mm and 2.6 mm, and working channel diameters of 1.2 mm and 0.5 mm, respectively, Olympus Medical Systems, Tokyo, Japan)[17] (**Fig. 1**A,B) and a video PTCS (ECN-1530, 5.3 mm outer diameter and 2 mm working channel; Pentax Co. Ltd, Tokyo, Japan) (**Fig. 2**A,B) are commercially available in Japan.

Image-enhanced cholangiopancreatoscopy techniques are being evaluated for use in pancreatobiliary diseases and in diseases of the gastrointestinal (GI) tract, including chromocholangioscopy with dye solution, autofluorescence imaging (AFI), and narrow-band imaging (NBI) in addition to conventional white light illumination. Preliminary clinical experience suggests that these innovative enhanced imaging techniques may help distinguish benign from malignant diseases, and highlight certain features such as mucosal structures and mucosal microvessels. This article summarizes the

No conflicts of interest exist.
[a] Department of Gastroenterology and Hepatology, Tokyo Medical University, Nishishinjuku 6-7-1, Shinjuku-ku, Tokyo 160-0023, Japan
[b] Department of Internal Medicine, Evangelisches Krankenhaus Düsseldorf, Kirchfeldstrasse 40, 40217 Düsseldorf, Germany
[c] Division of Gastroenterology & Hepatology University of Colorado Denver, MS F735, 1635 Aurora Court, Rm AIP 2.031, Aurora, CO 80045, USA
* Corresponding author.
E-mail address: itoi@tokyo-med.ac.jp (T. Itoi).

Gastrointest Endoscopy Clin N Am 19 (2009) 557–566
doi:10.1016/j.giec.2009.06.002
1052-5157/09/$ – see front matter © 2009 Elsevier Inc. All rights reserved.

Table 1
Typical cholangioscopy findings in benign and malignant bile ducts using WL, ME, NBI, and AFI

	WL	ME	NBI	AFI
Normal	Flat surface (+/− shallow pseudodiverticula)	Enhanced surface structure by blue staining	Enhanced surface structure and vessels	Light green
	Fine network of normal vessels	—	—	—
Inflammation	Bumpy surface, pseudodiverticula	Enhanced surface structure by blue staining	Enhanced surface structure and vessels	Light green, green
	Regular granular lesions (hyperplasia)	—	—	—
	Thin tortuous vessels	—	—	—
Scar	Convergence of folds, white mucosa	Enhanced surface structure by blue staining	Enhanced surface structure; paucity of vessels	Light green
Cancer	Irregularly papillary or granular lesions	No stained surface[a]	Enhanced surface structure and vessels	Green, dark green
	Nodular elevated lesions	—	—	—
	Thin to thick tortuous vessels	—	—	—

Abbreviations: AFI, autofluorescence imaging; ME, methylene blue stained imaging; NBI, narrow-band imaging; WL, white light imaging.
[a] When tumor surface is covered with mucin or exudates, false staining can be seen.

features of image-enhanced video cholangioscopy with dye solution, AFI, and NBI as novel diagnostic tools.

CHROMOCHOLANGIOSCOPY

In GI-tract diseases, it is well known that chromoendoscopy with various dyes enable delineation of the tumor margins. Chromoendoscopy using crystal violet, indigo carmine, or methylene blue is, reportedly, a helpful tool to distinguish neoplastic from non-neoplastic colonic polyps,[18,19] or malignancy in Barrett's esophagus.[20–22] Two studies evaluated the usefulness of fiberoptic peroral cholangioscopy (POCS) or PTCS in biliary-tract lesions, using 0.1% methylene blue for better observation.[23,24] At first, 0.1% methylene blue was instilled through the working channel. Excess dye was removed by suction after a waiting period of 2 minutes, and then the lesions were observed during continuous irrigation of saline solution through the working channel.[24] Maetani and colleagues[23] described different methylene blue staining properties related to types of biliary epithelia—normal, metaplasia, or cancer—by

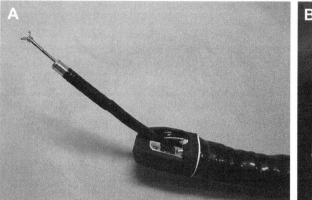
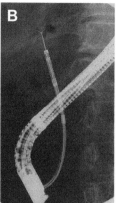

Fig.1. Mother-and-baby–type peroral video cholangioscopy system. (*A*) In this system, a miniature biopsy forceps (diameter: 1 mm) can be advanced through the working channel (diameter: 1.2 mm) of a peroral video cholangioscope (CHF-B260, Olympus Medical Systems). (*B*) Radiograph of duodenoscope with a peroral cholangioscope and biopsy forceps in the bile duct.

correlating the histologic analysis of frozen sections with forceps biopsy specimens obtained during PTCS. They reported that cancerous epithelia stained significantly less often than either normal or metaplastic epithelia. Hoffman and colleagues[24] reported that with POCS, neoplastic findings showed irregular mucosa with inhomogeneous and intensively dark-blue staining patterns, whereas non-neoplastic findings had a smooth surface mucosa with homogeneous staining. However, Maetani and colleagues[23] suggested that blue epithelium seen on chromocholangioscopy is not always truly epithelium stained by methylene blue, because the endoscopic findings sometimes differed from the microscopic findings. The main reason for this discrepancy is that methylene blue adhered to mucus or exudate on the surface of the biliary epithelium. The authors reported an initial experience with video PTCS (ECN-1530, 5 mm outer diameter and 2 mm working channel, Pentax Co. Ltd) using methylene blue in the same way (see **Table 1**).[25] Video chromocholangioscopy displayed more

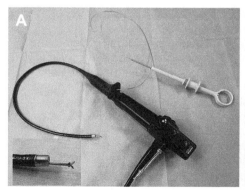
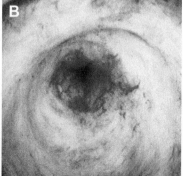

Fig. 2. Percutaneous transhepatic video cholangioscopy. (*A*) Dedicated percutaneous transhepatic video cholangioscope (outer diameter: 5.3 mm, working channel diameter: 2.0 mm, ECN-1530, Pentax Co. Ltd). (*B*) Endoscopic imaging of bile duct cancer by PTCS.

details of the mucosal structure than conventional PTCS. However, regardless of whether the lesion was neoplastic, vessels became unclear owing to surrounding dark-blue staining. Interestingly, chromocholangioscopy revealed many rounded dimple lesions, or shallow pseudodiverticula, in some non-neoplastic bile ducts (**Fig. 3**). We call these round dimpled lesions "the dimple sign" and they are indicative of non-neoplastic bile duct histology.

Brauer and colleagues[26] published an initial report using video POCS with indigo carmine in a patient with intraductal papillary mucinous neoplasm of the bile duct. Bile duct irrigation with acetylcysteine solution was first performed before tissue staining to help dislodge the thick mucin material. Although chromocholangioscopy has some potential for enhancing visualization of bile duct lesions, the presence of mucus, exudate, bile, or contrast tends to obscure mucosal details and often interferes with the ability to achieve adequate tissue staining.

AUTOFLUORESCENCE CHOLANGIOSCOPY

The authors evaluated the usefulness of AFI in patients with biliary-tract diseases using a laser-induced, fluorescence endoscopy-GI system (LIFE-GI, Xillix Technologies Corp, Vancouver, British Columbia, Canada) or a system of autofluorescence endoscopy (SAFE, Pentax Co. Ltd).[25] Fiberoptic PTCS (FCN-15X: 5.0 mm outer diameter and 2.0 mm working channel, Pentax Co. Ltd; CHF-P20: 4.9 mm outer diameter and 2.2 mm working channel, Olympus Medical Systems) or fiberoptic POCS (FCP-9P, 3.0 mm outer diameter and 1.2 mm working channel, Pentax Co. Ltd) were used in the LIFE-GI system. In the AFI mode, blue excitation light is first delivered to the bile duct through the light guide of a fiberoptic cholangioscope. Autofluorescence light is then detected by two hypersensitive green field and red field cameras. After manipulating those imaging signals, normal mucosa is green but neoplastic lesions change from green to dark green or black owing to differences in the intensity of the autofluorescence (see **Table 1**). To obtain better images, saline solution was used for continuous irrigation.

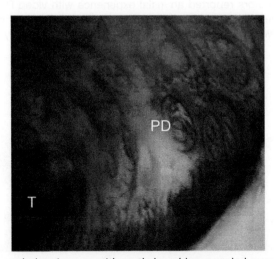

Fig. 3. Video chromocholangioscopy with methylene blue revealed many rounded dimple lesions (PD) in the bile duct around malignant stricture (T) which appeared dark because methylene blue adhered to mucus or exudate on the surface of the neoplastic epithelium.

Sixty-five biliary tract lesions were examined to compare the diagnostic ability of conventional PTCS with or without AFI.[25] The diagnostic ability of conventional cholangioscopy without and with AFI are as follows: sensitivity 88% and 100%, specificity 87.5% and 52.5%, accuracy 87.7% and 70.8%, respectively. Interestingly, in three cases of bile duct cancer, AFI detected lateral cancer spread that was missed by conventional PTCS (**Fig. 4**). On the other hand, the frequency of false-positive results increased with AFI. Non-neoplastic granular mucosa tended to appear slightly dark green, and bile was recognized as dark-green fluid. During POCS, bile often hindered the field of view because saline irrigation is difficult to achieve through a small working channel. The authors agree with Uedo and colleagues[27] that the image quality of the fiberoptic endoscopes is not sufficient, resulting in low specificity. A dedicated AFI video cholangioscopy system may help to improve the diagnostic accuracy of AFI in the future.[28]

NBI

The newly developed NBI system (CV-260SL processor, CVL-260SL light source, Olympus Medical Systems) is based on the modification of spectral features with an optical color-separation filter narrowing the bandwidth of spectral transmittance.[29] The filter is placed in the optical illumination system. The filter eliminates all illumination wavelengths, except two narrow wavelengths. The central wavelengths of each band are 415 nm and 540 nm. The image is reproduced in the processor with information from two illumination bands. The wavelength of 415 nm provides the most information on the capillary and pit patterns of the superficial mucosa, and the wavelength of 540 nm provides information about thicker capillaries in slightly deeper tissues. The mode change is easily performed by pushing a button in the handle of the cholangioscope, and the switch occurs in 1 second. Two video cholangioendoscopes are available (CHF-B260 and CHF-BP260, Olympus Medical Systems).[17] Biopsies can be performed under direct vision using a 3-Fr diameter ultrathin biopsy forceps (FB-44U-1, Olympus Medical Systems); see **Fig. 1B**.

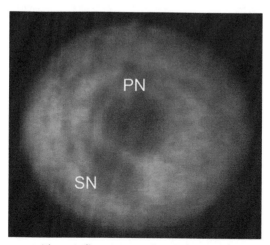

Fig. 4. Cholangioscopy with autofluorescence imaging. Normal mucosa is green but neoplastic lesions appear dark green or black owing to differences in the intensity of the autofluorescence. Autofluorescence imaging can detect not only the primary neoplasm (PN) but also delineate the outer limits of mucosal spreading neoplasm (SN).

In GI-tract diseases, NBI enhances visualization of fine surface mucosal structures and mucosal capillary microvessels compared with white light endoscopy.[28,30–34] There are pilot studies of endoscopic imaging of the pancreatobiliary system using NBI,[26,35–40] mostly involving a small number of cases.

NBI CHOLANGIOSCOPY

To evaluate the feasibility of the NBI system for clinical use, its ability to identify biliary tract lesions was compared with conventional observation. The evaluation points were (1) the delineation of the proximal or, possibly, distal margins and (2) identification of vessels on the surface of the lesions (see **Table 1**).[35]

Twenty-one lesions in 12 patients were evaluated using POCS with conventional white light imaging and NBI. In bile duct cancers, only the distal portion of the primary lesions was examined. In contrast, the proximal portion was evaluated in two cases in which POCS could traverse the tumor to the hepatic side. Regardless of benign or malignant etiology, the ability of NBI observation to identify both the surface structure and mucosal vessels was as good as, or better than, conventional observation (**Fig. 5**).[35] In particular, at the sites of superficial tumor spread, NBI tended to be better than conventional observation at detecting the lesion and delineating the margins.[35,37] These results suggest that video cholangioscopy may be helpful not only for differentiation between benign and malignant lesions but also for diagnosis of bile duct tumors showing superficial spread, such as papillary-growth–type bile duct cancer or intraductal papillary mucinous neoplasm (IPMN) of the bile duct.

NBI made it possible to detect more fine surface mucosal structures and microvessels than conventional POCS. Normal bile ducts showed a smooth surface, often accompanied by the dimple sign, as also seen on chromoendoscopy. Thin and regular mucosal capillary microvessels were seen frequently in normal bile ducts. Tiny hyperplastic changes were more obvious by NBI. NBI cholangioscopy has some technical challenges. One of the issues is that bile and blood both appear as dark red fluid in the

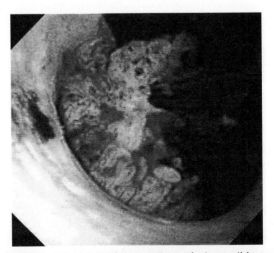

Fig. 5. Peroral video cholangioscopy with NBI. NBI made it possible to detect more fine surface mucosal structures and microvessels than with white light imaging. However, bile and blood are recognized as dark red fluid in the NBI mode, which can obscure some mucosal details.

NBI mode. The other is that, unlike endoscopes for the GI tract, the current cholangio-scope is not equipped with a magnifying system.

NBI PANCREATOSCOPY

Video peroral pancreatoscopy (POPS) can play a similar role as POCS. However, with POPS one of the greatest issues is scope insertion because the standard cholangio-scope is 3.1 to 3.4 mm; whereas the smallest diameter POPS (CHF-BP260, Olympus Medical Systems) is 2.6 mm but has no biopsy capabilities. The indications for POPSs, therefore, are limited. IPMN is a good indication for performing POPS, both to delineate the extent of duct involvement and to assess benign versus malignant features. Main-duct IPMN is particularly amenable to POPS because of a patulous papilla and enlarged pancreatic duct.

Some reports described, the POPS scope has been successfully inserted into the main pancreatic duct and reached the pancreas tail using a guidewire without any early or late procedure-related complications.[36,41] The authors evaluated 14 lesions in 9 patients using POPS with conventional white light imaging and NBI. Regardless of benign or malignant etiology, the ability of NBI observation to identify both the surface structure and mucosal vessels was as good as, or better than, conventional observation.[41]

LIMITATIONS

Since peroral video cholangiopancreatoscopes are very long and ultrathin, and have to navigate multiple loops and turns, their maneuverability and fragility are the greatest issues. Moreover, current cholangiopancreatoscopes are not equipped with magnification. Although video PTCS has better endoscopic imaging and good maneuverability because of its shorter length, percutaneous transhepatic approach has some drawbacks: (1) the necessity of long hospitalization, (2) cumbersome management of a drainage catheter, and (3) serious complications including bleeding, seeding metastasis along the sinus tract of percutaneous transhepatic drainage, and risk of intraperitoneal metastasis.

With regard to the diagnostic value of enhanced imaging techniques, most published reports are pilot studies with relatively small numbers of patients, and the investigators were usually not blinded to the clinical data, which can influence the interpretation of images.

SUMMARY

Although some technical challenges still need to be overcome, image-enhanced cholangiopancratoscopy appears to be a promising modality to improve diagnostic accuracy of pancreatobiliary diseases. Large randomized double-blind studies are needed to confirm the diagnostic value of these promising advanced imaging technologies.

ACKNOWLEDGMENTS

The authors are indebted to Prof. J. Patrick Barron of the International Medical Communication Center of Tokyo Medical University for his review of this manuscript.

REFERENCES

1. Takekoshi T, Takagi K. Retrograde pancreatocholangioscopy [in Japanese with English abstract]. Gastroenterol Endosc 1975;17:678–83.
2. Nakajima M, Akasaka Y, Fukumoto K, et al. Peroral cholangiopancreatoscopy (PCPS) under duodenoscopic guidance. Am J Gastroenterol 1978;66:241–7.
3. Rösch W, Koch H, Demling L. Peroral cholangioscopy. Endoscopy 1976;8: 172–5.
4. Kozarek R. Direct cholangioscopy and pancreatoscopy at time of endoscopic retrograde cholangiopancreatography. Am J Gastroenterol 1988;83:55–7.
5. Chen YK, Pleskow DK. Spyglass single-operator peroral cholangiopancreatoscopy system for the diagnosis and therapy of bile-duct disorders: a clinical feasibility study (with video). Gastrointest Endosc 2007;65:832–41.
6. Hara T, Yamaguchi T, Ishihara T, et al. Diagnosis and patients management of intraductal papillary-mucinous tumor of the pancreas by using peroral pancreatoscopy and intraductal ultrasonography. Gastroenterology 2002;122:34–43.
7. Yamao K, Ohashi K, Nakamura T, et al. Efficacy of peroral pancreatoscopy in the diagnosis of pancreatic diseases. Gastrointest Endosc 2003;57:205–9.
8. Neuhause H. Cholangioscopy. Endoscopy 1992;24:125–32.
9. Takada T, Suzuki S, Nakamura K, et al. Studies in percutaneous biliary tract endoscopy. Gastroenterol Endosc 1974;16:106–11.
10. Nimura Y, Shionoya S, Hayakawa N, et al. Value of percutaneous transhepatic cholangioscopy (PTCS). Surg Endosc 1988;2:213–9.
11. Seo DW, Lee SK, Yoo KS, et al. Cholangioscopic findings in bile duct tumors. Gastrointest Endosc 2000;52:630–4.
12. Sato M, Inoue H, Ogawa S, et al. Limitation of percutaneous transhepatic cholangioscopy for the diagnosis of the intramural extension of bile duct carcinoma. Endoscopy 1998;30:281–8.
13. Itoi T, Shinohara Y, Takeda K, et al. Detection of telomerase activity in biopsy specimens for diagnosis of biliary tract cancers. Gastrointest Endosc 2000;52: 380–6.
14. Meenan J, Schoeman M, Rauws E, et al. A video baby cholangioscope. Gastrointest Endosc 1995;42:584–5.
15. Kodama T, Koshitani T, Sato H, et al. Electronic pancreatoscopy for the diagnosis of pancreatic diseases. Am J Gastroenterol 2002;97:617–22.
16. Yasuda K, Sakata M, Ueda M, et al. The use of pancreatoscopy in the diagnosis of intraductal papillary mucinous tumor lesions of the pancreas. Clin Gastroenterol Hepatol 2005;3:S53–7.
17. Igarashi Y, Okano N, Sato D, et al. Peroral cholangioscopy using a new thinner videoscope (CHF-B260). Dig Endosc 2005;17:S63–6.
18. Konishi K, Kaneko K, Kurahashi T, et al. A comparison of magnifying and non-magnifying colonoscopy for diagnosis of colorectal polyps: a prospective study. Gastrointest Endosc 2002;57:48–53.
19. Fu KI, Sano Y, Kato S, et al. Chromoendoscopy using indigo carmine dye spraying with magnifying observation is the most reliable methods for differential diagnosis between non-neoplastic and neoplastic colorectal lesions: a prospective study. Endoscopy 2004;36:1089–93.
20. Horwhat JD, Maydonovitch CL, Ramos F, et al. A randomized comparison of methylene blue-directed biopsy versus conventional four-quadrant biopsy for the detection of intestinal metaplasia and dysplasia in patients with long-segment Barrett's esophagus. Am J Gastroenterol 2008;103:546–54.

21. Canto MI, Setrakian S, Willis J, et al. Methylene blue selectively stains intestinal metaplasia in Barrett's esophagus. Gastrointest Endosc 1996;44:1–7.
22. Amano Y, Kushiyama Y, Ishihara S, et al. Crystal violet chromoendoscopy with mucosal pit pattern diagnosis is useful for surveillance of short-segment Barrett's esophagus. Am J Gastroenterol 2005;100:21–6.
23. Maetani I, Ogawa S, Sato M, et al. Lack of methylene blue staining in superficial epithelia as a possible marker for superficial lateral spread of bile duct cancer. Diagn Ther Endosc 1996;3:29–34.
24. Hoffman A, Kiesslich R, Bittinger F, et al. Methylene blue-aided cholangioscopy in patients with biliary strictures: feasibility and outcome analysis. Endoscopy 2008; 40:563–71.
25. Itoi T, Shinohara S, Takeda K, et al. Improvement of choledochoscopy-chromoendoscopy, autofluorescense imaging, or narrow-band imaging. Dig Endosc 2007; 19:S95–102.
26. Brauer BC, Fukami N, Chen YK. Direct cholangioscopy with narrow-band imaging, chromoendoscopy, and argon plasma coagulation of intraductal papillary mucinous neoplasm of the bile duct (with videos). Gastrointest Endosc 2008; 67:574–6.
27. Uedo N, Ishii H, Tatsuta M, et al. A novel videoendoscopy system by using autofluorescence and reflectance imaging for diagnosis of esophagogastric cancers. Gastrointest Endosc 2005;62:521–8.
28. Kara MA, Bergman JJ. Autofluorescence imaging and narrow-band imaging for the detection of early neoplasia in patients with Barrett's esophagus. Endoscopy 2006;38:627–31.
29. Gono K, Yamazaki K, Doguchi N, et al. Endoscopic observation of tissue by narrowband illumination. Opt Rev 2003;10:211–5.
30. Nakayoshi T, Tajiri H, Matsuda K, et al. Magnifying endoscopy combined with narrow band imaging system for early gastric cancer: correlation of vascular pattern with histopathology. Endoscopy 2004;36:1080–4.
31. Yoshida T, Inoue H, Usui S, et al. Narrow-band imaging system with magnifying endoscopy for superficial esophageal lesions. Gastrointest Endosc 2004;59: 288–95.
32. Machida T, Sano Y, Hamamoto Y, et al. Narrow-band imaging in the diagnosis of colorectal mucosal lesions: a pilot study. Endoscopy 2004;36:1094–8.
33. Kara MA, Ennahachi M, Fockens P, et al. Detection and classification of the mucosal and vascular patterns (mucosal morphology) in Barrett's esophagus by using narrow band imaging. Gastrointest Endosc 2006;64:155–66.
34. Hirata M, Tanaka S, Oka S, et al. Evaluation of microvessels in colorectal tumors by narrow band imaging magnification. Gastrointest Endosc 2007;66:945–52.
35. Itoi T, Sofuni A, Itokawa F, et al. Peroral cholangioscopic diagnosis of biliary tract diseases using narrow-band imaging. Gastrointest Endosc 2007;66:730–6.
36. Itoi T, Sofuni A, Itokawa F, et al. Initial experience of peroral pancreatoscopy combined with narrow-band imaging in diagnosis of intraductal papillary mucinous neoplasms of the pancreas. Gastrointest Endosc 2007;66:793–7.
37. Lu XL, Itoi T, Kubota K. Cholangioscopy using narrow band imaging and transpapillary radiotherapy for mucin-producing bile duct tumor. Clin Gastroenterol Hepatol 2009;7:e34–5.
38. Itoi T, Sofuni A, Itokawa F, et al. What's new on the cholangioscopy? Is narrow-band imaging cholangioscopy next generation? Dig Endosc 2007;19:S87–94.
39. Tanaka K, Yasuda K, Uno K, et al. Evaluation of narrow band imaging for peroral cholangiopancratoscopy. Dig Endosc 2007;19:S129–33.

40. Igarashi Y, Okano N, Ito K, et al. Endoscopic observation of mucosal spread lesion of cholangiocarcinoma using peroral cholangioscopy with narrow band imaging. Dig Endosc 2007;19:S109–14.

41. Itoi T, Sofuni A, Itokawa F. Diagnosis of pancreaticobiliary diseases using cholangioscopy and pancreatoscopy with narrow-band imaging. In: Niwa H, Tajiri H, Nakajima M, Yasuda K, editors. New challenges in gastrointestinal endoscopy. New York: Springer; 2008. p. 466–71.

Cholangiopancreatoscopy for Targeted Biopsies of the Bile and Pancreatic Ducts

Shahzad Iqbal, MD[a], Peter D. Stevens, MD[a,b],*

KEYWORDS

- Cholangioscopy • Pancreatoscopy • ERCP
- Biliary stricture • Pancreatic stricture • Intraductal endoscopy
- Directed biopsy • Image-guided biopsy

With the advances in intra-abdominal imaging, there has been a shift from diagnostic to therapeutic endoscopic retrograde cholangiopancreatography (ERCP). The use of ERCP as a pure diagnostic test has significantly diminished. Nonetheless, ERCP maintains the advantage over intra-abdominal imaging in that it offers access to the pancreatobiliary system for tissue diagnosis. Standard ERCP-sampling techniques reliant on fluoroscopic imaging, however, have low-to-moderate sensitivity for pancreatobiliary cancer detection.[1,2] Intraductal endoscopic visualization of the biopsy target during peroral cholangioscopy (POC) or peroral pancreatoscopy (POP) might enhance the diagnostic value of ERCP by improving target selection and tissue acquisition.

In this article, the authors describe POC- and POP-sampling techniques and their contribution to the diagnosis of pancreatobiliary diseases. A Pubmed search was conducted to identify all relevant publications on image-guided biopsy technique. The key words used were: peroral cholangioscopy, peroral choledochoscopy, peroral pancreatoscopy, intraductal endoscopy, SpyGlass, directed biopsy, image-guided biopsy, and SpyBite-forceps biopsy. The yield of standard non-image–guided ERCP-sampling techniques is reviewed first, followed by detailed description of image-guided sampling techniques.

NON-IMAGE–GUIDED TISSUE-SAMPLING TECHNIQUES

Standard techniques were analyzed for malignant biliary stricture in two review articles by de Bellis and colleagues.[1,2] These consist of either intraductal fluid aspiration

[a] Division of Digestive and Liver Diseases, Department of Medicine, Columbia University College of Physicians and Surgeons, P&S 10-508, 630 West 168th Street, NY 10032, USA
[b] Columbia University Medical Center, New York Presbyterian Hospital, Irving Pavilion, 8th Floor, 161 Fort Washington Avenue, NY 10032, USA
* Corresponding author. Columbia University Medical Center, New York Presbyterian Hospital, Irving Pavilion, 8th Floor, 161 Fort Washington Avenue, NY 10032, USA.
E-mail address: Pds5@columbia.edu (P.D. Stevens).

Gastrointest Endoscopy Clin N Am 19 (2009) 567–577
doi:10.1016/j.giec.2009.06.005
1052-5157/09/$ – see front matter © 2009 Published by Elsevier Inc.

cytology, cytologic-histologic analysis of retrieved plastic stents, fine-needle–aspiration (FNA) cytology, brush cytology, endobiliary forceps biopsy (**Table 1**), or combination of above.

Although the specificity was almost 100% with the above techniques, the sensitivity was low-to-moderate. The most effective method for obtaining tissue diagnosis was combining two or more techniques. Combining one cytologic method with forceps biopsy was more often diagnostic.[3] The cancer detection rate varied from 55% to 73% with the combination of biopsy and brushings; and 62% to 82% with the combination of biopsy, brushings, and fine-needle aspiration.[2] The authors, however, concluded that multimodal sampling was more time-consuming and technically difficult when compared with the use of a single technique.

The yield is even lower for pancreatic malignancy, as shown in **Table 2**. The single best technique was the use of forceps biopsy for ampullary cancer, with a detection rate of 77% to 88%.[3] These findings are logical as ampullary malignancy can be visualized endoscopically and sampled directly.

IMAGE-GUIDED TISSUE-SAMPLING TECHNIQUES
Biliary Malignancy

In the setting of biliary malignancy, cholangioscopy can be used for the visual diagnosis of malignancy by assessing for the typical features including "tumor vessels" (ie, irregularly dilated and tortuous vessels), intraductal nodules or masses, infiltrative or ulcerated strictures, and papillary or villous mucosal projections.[4,5] The sensitivity of cholangioscopy is further improved by directed biopsies. In a study by Kim and colleagues,[6] the presence of tumor vessels had a sensitivity of 61% but, when combined with percutaneous biopsy, diagnosed 96% of cancers. In **Table 3**, all studies on image-guided sampling for biliary malignancy have been mentioned in chronologic order.

In a study by Langer and colleagues,[7] 64 cholangiopancreatoscopic procedures were performed in 52 consecutive patients by using Olympus BP30, Olympus video CHFB160, and Pentax FCP9P scopes. Cholangioscopic biopsy was obtained in 26 patients using a prototype Olympus biopsy forceps. Fourteen patients had confirmed malignancies: seven by cholangiopancreatography (CP) with cholangioscopic forceps biopsy (CFB), five visualized by CP, and two intraoperatively. The sensitivity for cancer detection was 85.7%. The authors concluded that CFB improved the ability of CP to confirm malignancy.

Fukuda and colleagues[8] studied the utility of POC for distinguishing malignant from benign biliary disease. A total of 97 consecutive patients (76 strictures and 21 filling defects), were included in the study. Standard-type Olympus peroral cholangioscopes (CHF-B20, 4.5 mm diameter; CHF-BP30, 3.4 mm diameter; CHF-B260, 3.1 mm diameter; Olympus) were used. Brushing cytology or endobiliary forceps biopsy also was performed. ERCP-tissue sampling correctly identified 22 of 38 malignant strictures and all 35 benign lesions except in three patients with inadequate samples (accuracy, 78.0%; sensitivity, 57.9%; specificity, 100%; positive predictive value [PPV] 100%; negative predictive value [NPV] 68.6%). The addition of POC correctly identified all 38 malignant strictures and 33 of 38 benign lesions (accuracy, 93.4%; sensitivity, 100%; specificity, 86.8%; PPV 88.45; NPV 100%). For the 21 filling defects observed by ERCP, POC correctly diagnosed all 8 malignant diseases and 13 benign lesions (accuracy 94.8%; sensitivity 100%; specificity 90.2%; PPV 90.2%; NPV 100%). The authors concluded that the addition of POC to tissue sampling improves the diagnostic ability and covers for insufficient sensitivity. POC was especially useful for diagnosing a filling defect.

Table 1
Non-image–guided tissue sampling techniques for biliary malignancy

Technique	References	Number of Patients	Number of Cancers	True Positives	Sensitivity	Specificity	Positive Predictive Value	Negative Predictive Value
Bile aspirate	6[24-29]	351	281	76	27%	100%	100%	25%
Retrieved stent	6[24,29-33]	197	145	50	34%	100%	100%	35%
FNA	5[3,34-37]	223	187	62	34%	100%	100%	22%
Brush cytology	8[3,24,29,38-42]	837	578	241	42%	98%	9%	43%
Forceps biopsy	6[3,28,39,40,43,44]	502	343	191	56%	97%	97%	51%

Data from de Bellis M, Sherman S, Fogel EL, et al. Tissue sampling at ERCP in suspected malignant biliary strictures (Part 1). Gastrointest Endosc 2002;56(4): 522–61; and de Bellis M, Sherman S, Fogel EL, et al. Tissue sampling at ERCP in suspected malignant biliary strictures (Part 2). Gastrointest Endosc 2002;56(5):720–30.[1,2]

Table 2
Non-image–guided tissue sampling techniques for pancreatic malignancy

Technique	Number of Studies	Number of Cancers	True Positive	Sensitivity
Brush cytology	9[28,29,37,39–42,45,46]	202	75	37%
FNA	1[3]	46	14	30%
Forceps biopsy	6[3,28,39,40,43,45]	90	44	49%

Data from de Bellis M, Sherman S, Fogel EL, et al. Tissue sampling at ERCP in suspected malignant biliary strictures (Part 1). Gastrointest Endosc 2002;56(4):552–61.[1]

Shah and colleagues[9] reported the usefulness of cholangioscopy in patients with indeterminate pancreaticobiliary pathology. Sixty-two consecutive patients during a period of 2.5 years underwent cholangioscopy followed by either cholangioscopy-directed (obtained under direct-visualization) or cholangioscopy-assisted (obtained through duodenoscope) biopsies. The following cholangioscopes were used: Olympus BP30 (fiberoptic), Pentax FCP9P (fiberoptic; Pentax, Orangeburg, NY, USA), and Olympus CHF B160 (video). A minimum of three passes and bites were attempted with each biopsy method. Thirty-nine of 42 (93%) of the cholangioscopy-directed and all of the cholangioscopy-assisted biopsies were deemed to be adequate specimens for diagnosis. Sixteen of 18 (89%) patients with a final diagnosis of malignancy were detected. The two missed cancers were intrahepatic cholangiocarcinoma. The authors concluded that the cholangioscopy with and without biopsy was highly accurate in diagnosing and excluding pancreatobiliary malignancy in patients with indeterminate strictures.

Tischendorf and colleagues[10] considered the role of POC in 53 primary sclerosing cholangitis (PSC) patients with dominant bile duct stenoses. In this study, 53 patients underwent POC and endoscopic tissue sampling (biopsy or brush cytology) in addition to ERCP. Transpapillary cholangioscopy was performed using a cholangioscope with an outer diameter of 2.97 mm (9 Fr) (2D-Microendoscope ERCP, 180 cm long, Almikro Ltd, Bad Krozingen, Germany). Twelve patients (23%) had dominant bile duct stenoses caused by cholangiocarcinoma, whereas 41 of the 53 patients (77%) had benign dominant bile duct stenoses. Cholangioscopy (with and without tissue sampling) was significantly superior to ERCP for detecting malignancy in terms of its sensitivity (92% vs 66%; $P = .25$), specificity (93% vs 51%; $P<.001$), accuracy (93% vs 55%; $P<.001$), PPV (79% vs 29%; $P<.001$), and NPV (97% vs 84%; $P<.001$). The authors concluded that transpapillary cholangioscopy significantly increased the ability to distinguish between malignant and benign dominant bile duct stenoses in patients with PSC.

Chen and Pleskow[11] evaluated the clinical utility and safety of the SpyGlass peroral cholangiopancreatoscopy system (SpyGlass Direct Visualization System; Microvasive Endoscopy, Boston Scientific Corp, Natick, MA, USA) for diagnostic and therapeutic endoscopic procedures in bile ducts. SpyGlass procedures were performed in 35 patients: 22 with indeterminate strictures (63%), 5 with indeterminate filling defects (14%), 5 with stones (14%), 2 with cystic lesions (6%), and 1 patient with an indication for gallbladder stent placement (3%). The rate of procedural success was 91% (95% confidence interval 77%–98%). Twenty patients underwent SpyGlass-directed biopsy, and the specimens obtained from 19 patients (95%) were found adequate for histologic evaluation. Median bites and specimens per patient were five and four and a half, respectively. The preliminary sensitivity and specificity of SpyGlass-directed biopsy to diagnose malignancy were 71% and 100%, respectively. The authors concluded that the SpyGlass procedure is clinically feasible and provided adequate samples for histologic diagnosis.

Table 3
Image-guided sampling technique for biliary malignancy

Author	Year	Type	Number of Patients	Number of Cancers	True Positive	Sensitivity	Specificity	PPV	NPV
Langer [7]	2002	Pros	26	14	12	85.7%	100%	100%	85.7%
Fukuda [8]	2005	Pros	76	38	38	100%	86.8%	88.4%	100%
Shah [9]	2006	Pros	62	18	16	89%	96%	89%	96%
Tischendorf [10]	2006	Pros	53	12	11	92%	93%	79%	97%
Chen [11]	2007	Pros	20	7	5	71%	100%	100%	86.7%
Total			237	89	82	92%	93.2%	89%	95.2%

Abbreviation: Pros: prospective.

All the above studies were prospective in nature. The total number of patients was 237. Considering all the studies together, the cancer detection rate of image-guided sampling techniques for biliary malignancy was: sensitivity 92%, specificity 93.2%, PPV 89%, NPV 95.2%. Hence, the cancer detection rate is much higher than the previously described various non-image–guided sampling techniques (56% for forceps biopsy; and 62%–82% for biopsy, brushings, and FNA combined).

Pancreatic Malignancy

In the setting of pancreatic malignancy, pancreatoscopy guides tissue sampling by assessing for the presence of coarse mucosa, submucosal protrusion, friability, tumor vessel, and fish-egg–like and papillary projections.[12,13] The sensitivity and specificity of fish-egg–like, villous, and prominent mucosal protrusions is 68% and 87%, respectively.[14] Pancreatoscopic-guided tissue sampling greatly improves the diagnosis rate as compared with conventional tissue sampling. In a retrospective study of 11 patients with carcinoma in situ of the pancreas by Uehara and colleagues,[15] the diagnostic rate was 100% for pancreatoscopic cytology as compared with 60% for conventional pancreatic juice cytology. In **Table 4**, all studies on image-guided sampling for pancreatic malignancy have been mentioned in chronologic order.

The study by Yamaguchi and colleagues[16] comprised of 103 patients with intraductal papillary mucinous neoplasms (IPMN) who underwent surgical resection of pancreatic tumors (adenoma in 29 patients, borderline in17 patients, carcinoma in situ in 25 patients, and invasive carcinoma in 32 patients). Pancreatic juice was collected with a catheter after intravenous secretin injection in 71 patients and by POP in 32 patients. POP was done using mother-baby method: TJF10 scope (Olympus Optical) as mother, and BP-30 as baby scope. The sensitivity for IPMN was higher when pancreatic juice was collected by POP than by catheter (68.2% vs 38.2%; $P = 0.05$). The authors concluded that POP was useful for the collection of pancreatic juice in malignant IPMNs.

The study by Yasuda and colleagues[17] included 30 patients with IPMN who were resected and confirmed histologically. Among them, there were 6 cases of adenocarcinoma, 20 cases of adenoma, and 4 cases of hyperplasia. The pancreatoscope used was an electronic baby scope, which had a working channel for the forceps and a diameter of 3 mm. This model had up and down functions. POP was performed in 26 cases and characteristic findings such as a papillary tumor, redness, and proliferation of blood vessels, or fish-egg–like appearance were observed in 19 lesions. Among them, a papillary tumor was observed in eight cases, including 6 of 6 cases of adenocarcinoma and 2 of 16 cases of adenoma. The sensitivity for the detection of polypoid lesions greater than 3 mm compared with histology was 67% by POP, 92% by endoscopic ultrasound, and 100% by intraductal ultrasound. Eleven cases had POP-guided forceps biopsy, while POP-guided pancreatic fluid cytology was done in 18 cases. The sensitivity, specificity, PPV, and NPV of POP-guided biopsy and cytology were: 50% per 50%; 100% per 100%; 100% per 89%; and 62.5% per 87.5%, respectively. Other than tumor size and POP-directed biopsy examination, no other feature was capable of distinguishing adenomas from carcinomas. The authors concluded that POP is a useful method to evaluate IPMN, although there are some limitations in the accuracy and ability to perform a biopsy examination.

The authors found a paucity of studies on image-guided sampling techniques for pancreatic malignancy. All the above studies are retrospective in nature. The total number of patients is 61. By considering together all the above studies, the cancer detection rate was: sensitivity 62.5%, specificity 100%, PPV 100%, and NPV 70.7%. Although the cancer detection rate of image-guided sampling was lower for

Table 4
Image-guided sampling technique for pancreatic malignancy

Author	Year	Type	Number of Patients	Number of Cancers	True Positive	Sensitivity	Specificity	PPV	NPV
Yamaguchi[16]	2005	Retro	103	32	15	68.2%	100%	100%	58.8%
Yasuda[17] (pancreatic biopsy)	2005	Retro	11	6	3	50%	100%	100%	62.5%
Yasuda[41] (pancreatic cytology)	2005	Retro	18	4	2	50%	96%	89%	87.5%
Total			61	32	20	62.5%	100%	100%	70.7%

Abbreviation: Retro: retrospective.

pancreatic malignancy as compared with those for biliary malignancy (92%), it was still much higher as compared with non-image–guided sampling for pancreatic malignancy (30% for FNA, 37% for brushings, and 49% for biopsy).

IMPROVING IMAGE-GUIDED SAMPLING TECHNIQUE

Although intraductal endoscopy has enabled better a cancer detection rate for different pancreatobiliary malignancies, cancer detection still remains challenging in certain high-risk cases such as cholangiocarcinoma in PSC patients and pancreatic adenocarcinoma.

The recently described SpyGlass peroral CP system (SpyGlass Direct Visualization System; Microvasive Endoscopy, Boston Scientific Corp, Natick, MA, USA) has improved intraductal access and biopsy success rate. It is a single-operator–dependent system with four-way deflected steering and separate, dedicated irrigation channels.[18] In the porcine model, 14 SpyGlass-directed biopsies were performed above and 20 below the hepatic bifurcation. Adequate gross specimen was secured in 31 of 34 bites (91%). For purposes of histologic examination, the quality of 28 of 31 specimens (90%) was rated excellent to adequate.[18] In an initial human nonrandomized study of 35 patients by Chen and Pleskow,[11] 20 patients underwent SpyGlass-directed biopsy. The specimens procured from 19 patients (95%) were found adequate for histologic evaluation. Median bites and specimens per patient were five and four and a half, respectively. However, there is a need to improve this system. The fiberoptic images obtained with the SpyGlass System have quality that is inferior to that of digital images.[19] The development of a digital SpyGlass System incorporating charge-coupled device chip technology will overcome this deficit. This topic is discussed in detail in a separate article on the SpyGlass System by Chen and colleagues in this issue.

The cancer detection rate can also be improved by techniques that allow better visualization of the lesion such as narrow-band imaging (NBI). NBI has been shown to provide better visualization of vascular pattern and tumor vessels than conventional white light.[20,21] Techniques that image the lesion at microscopic level (eg, optical coherence tomography[22]) and confocal microscopy allow improved cancer diagnosis. In a study by Meining and colleagues,[23] targeted biopsies were taken in 14 patients with biliary strictures after mucosal imaging with a miniaturized, confocal laser-scanning miniprobe introduced by way of the accessory channel of a cholangioscope (Karl Storz, Tuttlingen, Germany). Presence of a black or dark-grey background with irregular, large white streaks (blood vessels filled with fluorescein) enabled prediction of neoplasia with an accuracy rate of 86%, sensitivity of 83%, and specificity of 88%. Hence, incorporation of technologies like NBI and confocal microscopy into the SpyGlass System will further enhance cancer detection rates.

SUMMARY

Intraductal POC- and POP-sampling techniques appear to offer an advantage over fluoroscopy-guided ERCP sampling techniques for the diagnosis of pancreatobiliary lesions. For biliary malignancy, the cancer detection rates with peroral cholangioscopic biopsy are: sensitivity 92%, specificity 93.2%, PPV 89%, and NPV 95.2%. The specimen adequacy rate is also higher ($\geq$90%) with peroral cholangioscopic forceps biopsy. Although the cancer detection rate is also higher with peroral pancreatoscopic sampling (sensitivity 62.5%, specificity 100%, PPV 100%, NPV 70.7%), there is a paucity of studies and larger prospective studies are needed. The authors believe that the cancer detection rate can be further improved in technically challenging cases by techniques offering better visualization such as NBI, optical coherence tomography, confocal microscopy, and further modifications of sampling tools.

REFERENCES

1. de Bellis M, Sherman S, Foel EL, et al. Tissue sampling at ERCP in suspected malignant biliary strictures (Part 1). Gastrointest Endosc 2002;56(4):552–61.
2. de Bellis M, Sherman S, Fogel EL, et al. Tissue sampling at ERCP in suspected malignant biliary strictures (Part 2). Gastrointest Endosc 2002;56(5):720–30.
3. Jailwala J, Fogel EL, Sherman S, et al. Triple tissue sampling at ERCP in malignant biliary obstruction. Gastrointest Endosc 2000;51:383–90.
4. Seo DW, Lee SK, Yoo KS, et al. Cholangioscopic findings in bile duct tumors. Gastrointest Endosc 2000;52:630–4.
5. Murata T, Nagasaka T, Kamiya J, et al. P53 labeling index in cholangioscopic biopsies is useful for determining spread of bile duct carcinomas. Gastrointest Endosc 2002;56:688–95.
6. Kim HJ, Kim MH, Lee SK, et al. Tumor vessel: a valuable cholangioscopic clue of malignant biliary stricture. Gastrointest Endosc 2000;52:635–8.
7. Langer DA, Shah RJ, Chen YK. The role of cholangiopancreatography (CP) and cholangioscopic forceps biopsy (CFB) in the management of pancreatobiliary (PB) diseases [abstract]. Gastrointest Endosc 2002;55(2):93.
8. Fukuda Y, Tsuyuguchi T, Sakai Y, et al. Diagnostic utility of peroral cholangioscopy for various bile-duct lesions. Gastrointest Endosc 2005;62:374–82.
9. Shah RJ, Langer DA, Antillon MR, et al. Cholangioscopy and cholangioscopic forceps biopsy in patients with indeterminate pancreaticobiliary pathology. Clin Gastroenterol Hepatol 2006;4:219–25.
10. Tischendorf JJ, Kruger M, Trautwein C, et al. Cholangioscopic characterization of dominant bile duct stenoses in patients with primary sclerosing cholangitis. Endoscopy 2006;38:665–9.
11. Chen YK, Pleskow DK. SpyGlass single-operator per oral cholangiopancreatoscopy system for the diagnosis and therapy of bile-duct disorders: a clinical feasibility study (with video). Gastrointest Endosc 2007;65:832–41.
12. Yamao K, Ohashi K, Nakamura T, et al. Efficacy of peroral pancreatoscopy in the diagnosis of pancreatic diseases. Gastrointest Endosc 2003;57:205–9.
13. Kodama T, Imamura Y, Sato H, et al. Feasibility study using a new small electronic pancreatoscope: description of findings in chronic pancreatitis. Endoscopy 2003;35:305–10.
14. Hara T, Yamaguchi T, Ishihara T, et al. Diagnosis and patient management of intraductal papillary mucinous tumor of the pancreas by using peroral pancreatoscopy and intraductal ultrasonography. Gastroenterology 2002;122:34–43.
15. Uehara H, Nakaizumi A, Tatsuta M, et al. Diagnosis of carcinoma in situ of the pancreas by peroral pancreatoscopy and pancreatoscopic cytology. Cancer 1997;79(3):454–61.
16. Yamaguchi T, Shirai Y, Ishihara T, et al. Pancreatic juice cytology in the diagnosis of intraductal papillary mucinous neoplasm of the pancreas: significance of sampling by peroral pancreatoscopy. Cancer 2005;104(12):2830–6.
17. Yasuda K, Sakata M, Ueda M, et al. The use of pancreatoscopy in the diagnosis of intraductal papillary mucinous tumor lesions of the pancreas. Clin Gastroenterol Hepatol 2005;7(Suppl 1):S53–7.

18. Chen YK. Preclinical characterization of the Spyglass peroral cholangiopancrea-toscopy system for direct access, visualization and biopsy. Gastrointest Endosc 2007;65:303–11.
19. Draganov P. The SpyGlass direct visualization system for cholangioscopy. J Gastroenterol Hepatol 2008;4(7):469–70.
20. Itoi T, Sofuni A, Itokawa F, et al. Peroral cholangioscopic diagnosis of biliary-tract diseases by using narrow-band imaging (with videos). Gastrointest Endosc 2007; 66(4):730–6.
21. Tanaka K, Yasuda K, Uno K, et al. Evaluation of narrow band imaging for peroral cholangiopancreatoscopy. Digestive Endoscopy 2007;19(Suppl 1):S129–33.
22. Poneros JM, Tearney GJ, Shiskov M, et al. Optical coherence tomography of the biliary tree during ERCP. Gastrointest Endosc 2002;55(1):84–8.
23. Meining A, Frimberger E, Becker V, et al. Detection of cholangiocarcinoma in vivo using miniprobe-based confocal fluorescence microscopy. Clin Gastroenterol Hepatol 2008;6(9):1057–60.
24. Foutch PG, Kerr DM, Harlan JR, et al. A prospective, controlled analysis of endoscopic cytotechniques for diagnosis of malignant biliary strictures. Am J Gastroenterol 1991;86:577–80.
25. Desa LA, Akosa AB, Lazzara S, et al. Cytodiagnosis in the management of extrahepatic biliary stricture. Gut 1991;32:1188–91.
26. Davidson B, Varsamidakis N, Dooley J, et al. Value of exfoliative cytology for investigating bile duct strictures. Gut 1992;33:1408–11.
27. Kurzawinski TR, Deery A, Dooley JS, et al. A prospective study of biliary cytology in 100 patients with bile duct strictures. Hepatology 1993;18:1399–403.
28. Sugiyama M, Atomi N, Wada N, et al. Endoscopic transpapillary bile duct biopsy without sphincterotomy for diagnosing biliary strictures: a prospective comparative study with bile and brush cytology. Am J Gastroenterol 1996;91:465–7.
29. Mansfield JC, Griffin SM, Wadebra V, et al. A prospective evaluation of cytology from biliary strictures. Gut 1997;49:671–7.
30. Leung JWC, Sung JY, Chung SCS, et al. Endoscopic scraping biopsy of malignant biliary strictures. Gastrointest Endosc 1989;35:65–6.
31. Pescatore P, Heubner C, Heine M, et al. The value of histological analysis of occluded biliary endoprostheses. Endoscopy 1995;27:597–600.
32. Simsir A, Greenebaum E, Stevens PD, et al. Biliary stent replacement cytology. Diagn Cytopathol 1997;16:233–7.
33. Deveraux B, Fogel E, Phillips S, et al. Biliary and pancreatic stent cytology in the diagnosis of pancreatobiliary malignancy [abstract]. Am J Gastroenterol 2000;95: 2475A.
34. Howell DA, Beveridge RP, Bosco J, et al. Endoscopic needle aspiration biopsy at ERCP in the diagnosis of biliary strictures. Gastrointest Endosc 1992;38:531–5.
35. Howell DA, Parsons WG, Jones MA, et al. Complete tissue sampling of biliary strictures at ERCP using a new device. Gastrointest Endosc 1996;43:498–501.
36. Lo SK, Cox J, Soltani S. A prospective blinded evaluation of all ERCP sampling methods on biliary strictures [abstract]. Gastrointest Endosc 1996;43:386A.
37. Farrell RJ, Jain AK, Brandwein SL, et al. The combination of stricture dilation, endoscopic needle aspiration and biliary brushings significantly improves diagnostic yield from malignant bile duct strictures. Gastrointest Endosc 2001;54: 587–94.
38. Lee JG, Leung JW, Baillie J, et al. Benign, dysplastic, or malignant—making sense of endoscopic bile duct brush cytology: results in 149 consecutive patients. Am J Gastroenterol 1995;90:722–6.

39. Ponchon T, Gagnon P, Berger F, et al. Value of endobiliary brush cytology and biopsies for the diagnosis of malignant bile duct stenosis: results of a prospective study. Gastrointest Endosc 1995;42:565–72.
40. Pugliese V, Conio M, Nicolò G, et al. Endoscopic retrograde forceps biopsy and brush cytology of biliary strictures: a prospective study. Gastrointest Endosc 1995;42:520–6.
41. Glasbrenner B, Ardan M, Boeck W, et al. Prospective evaluation of brush cytology of biliary strictures during endoscopic retrograde cholangiopancreatography. Endoscopy 1999;31:712–7.
42. Macken E, Drijkoningen M, Van Aken E, et al. Brush cytology of ductal strictures during ERCP. Acta Gastroenterol Belg 2000;63:254–9.
43. Kubota Y, Takaoka M, Tani K, et al. Endoscopic transpapillary biopsy for diagnosis of patients with pancreaticobiliary ductal strictures. Am J Gastroenterol 1993;88:1700–4.
44. Schoefl R, Haefner M, Wrba F, et al. Forceps biopsy and brush cytology during endoscopic retrograde cholangiopancreatography for the diagnosis of biliary stenoses. Scand J Gastroenterol 1997;32:363–8.
45. Wiersema M, Lehman G, Hawes R, et al. Improvement of diagnostic yield of brush cytology in malignant strictures by the use of supplemental tissue sampling technique [abstract]. Gastrointest Endosc 1992;35:265A.
46. Vandervoort J, Soetikno RM, Montes H, et al. Accuracy and complication rates of brush cytology from bile duct versus pancreatic duct. Gastrointest Endosc 1999;49:322–7.

Cholangioscopy for Special Applications: Primary Sclerosing Cholangitis, Liver Transplant, and Selective Duct Access

Bret T. Petersen, MD

KEYWORDS

- Cholangioscopy • Sclerosing cholangitis • Liver transplantation
- ERCP techniques • Cholangiocarcinoma

Endoscopic visualization of the gastrointestinal tract revolutionized gastroenterology. In contrast, cholangioscopy, or endoscopic access to the biliary and pancreatic ducts for direct visualization, was described more than 2 decades ago, but it did not generate enthusiasm for broad application until recently. Limitations included fragile and cumbersome cholangioscopes, the need for 2 endoscopists to perform cholangioscopic examinations, inadequate small caliber accessories, and absence of data demonstrating clinical benefit. During this time, endoscopic retrograde cholangiopancreatography (ERCP) evolved to become a predominantly therapeutic modality, often with concurrent intraductal tissue sampling. Despite widespread maturation of technical skills and improved device designs, ERCP techniques for sampling and for some therapies have fallen short of needs. Hence, the recent presentation of data demonstrating clinical benefit of cholangioscopy is generating renewed interest in its use for visually directed stone therapy, visual assessment of tissues, and targeted tissue sampling for diagnosis of neoplasia. Cholangioscopy is also being used for staging of the extent of mucosal-based lesions and occasionally for achieving difficult access to specific sections of the biliary or pancreatic ductal systems. This enthusiasm is also based on the availability of new cholangioscopes, including a single-operator partially disposable system (SpyGlass Direct Visualization System, Boston Scientific, Natick, MA, USA) and a prototype large image video chip endoscope (Olympus Corp, Tokyo), plus incorporation of narrow band imaging (NBI) capabilities

Department of Medicine, Division of Gastroenterology and Hepatology, Charlton 8, GI Endoscopy, Mayo Clinic, 200 First Street SW, Rochester, MN 55905, USA
E-mail address: petersen.bret@mayo.edu

Gastrointest Endoscopy Clin N Am 19 (2009) 579–586
doi:10.1016/j.giec.2009.06.003
1052-5157/09/$ – see front matter © 2009 Elsevier Inc. All rights reserved.

(CV-260SL processor, CVL-260SL Light Source, Olympus Corp) and enhanced accessories (eg, SpyBite Forceps, Boston Scientific).

This article addresses several challenging disease-specific or niche applications for which cholangioscopy holds some promise, including diagnostic and therapeutic use in patients with primary sclerosing cholangitis (PSC) and in those with complications following liver transplantation and use in gaining selective duct access when other means fail. Details regarding available cholangioscopes and devices and their use in general ERCP are provided elsewhere in this issue.

CHOLANGIOSCOPY IN PATIENTS WITH PSC

PSC is a chronic cholestatic disease characterized by the presence of fibrotic strictures of the intra- and extrahepatic biliary tree.[1] PSC typically culminates in cirrhosis and end-stage liver disease after 8 to 10 years. It is complicated by the development of symptomatic "dominant" strictures that contribute to jaundice, cholangitis, or stone formation in many patients and by cholangiocarcinoma in up to 10% to 30% of patients.[2] Identification of cholangiocarcinoma portends a poor diagnosis and significantly limits management options, as it is an absolute contraindication to liver transplantation, unless preceded by aggressive treatment regimens using combined radiation and chemotherapy as developed at the Mayo Clinic.[3]

The diagnosis of cholangiocarcinoma in the setting of PSC is challenging.[4] PSC-associated cholangiocarcinoma tends to present as obstruction of the large central ducts rather than as a parenchymal mass lesion from the peripheral ducts. Cholangiography is not specific and cannot distinguish malignant from benign lesions reliably.[5] Serum levels of carbohydrate antigen (CA) 19-9 are insensitive but potentially valuable for enhancing the suspicion of cholangiocarcinoma, in the absence of infectious cholangitis, pancreatitis, or pancreatic neoplasia, particularly when these levels are more than about 130 kU/L. Cross-sectional imaging with ultrasound has only low sensitivity for biliary cancer in PSC. Computed tomographic (CT) scanning can demonstrate secondary signs of ductal or vascular compromise, but infrequently localizes the tumor mass itself. Magnetic resonance imaging (MRI) with ferumoxide (Feridex) and gadolinium enhancement may be the single best modality for early investigation of possible cholangiocarcinoma.[4] Limited data are contradictory regarding the role of positron emission tomographic (PET) scanning for identification of cancer in PSC. ERCP for acquisition of tissue is central to the diagnosis of cholangiocarcinoma. Nevertheless, standard brush cytology and fluoroscopically guided intraductal biopsies are both insensitive (though highly specific). Advanced cytologic techniques using fluorescent in situ hybridization appear to significantly improve the sensitivity of cytologic diagnoses, at a small cost in specificity.[6]

In this setting, cholangioscopy has been investigated as a means toward more efficient diagnosis of cancer. In addition, recent data suggest that duct stones, particularly as identified by cholangioscopy, are much more common than previously realized.[7] Hence, with additional data, intraductal visualization may become a key modality in the management of patients with sclerosing cholangitis.

Awadallah and colleagues[7] from the University of Colorado reported the first consecutive series of procedures using cholangioscopy in patients with PSC for detection of duct stones or cholangiocarcinoma and for stone removal via cholangioscopically directed lithotripsy. Between 2000 and 2004, a prospective cohort of 41 patients with PSC underwent 60 procedures, including 55 via peroral ERCP access and 5 via percutaneous access. Antibiotic coverage and standard techniques were used. Various dedicated cholangioscopes with 1.2-mm operating channels and

3.1- to 3.4-mm external diameters were used from several manufacturers (Olympus fiberoptic, n = 50; Olympus digital video, n = 4; Pentax fiberoptic, n = 6). Of the 41 patients, 35 were evaluated for characterization of known dominant strictures, 1 for stone removal, and 4 for both concerns. Most patients presented with recurrent cholangitis (30) or worsening levels of liver enzymes (8). A large number of prior examinations had been performed, including a mean of 2.9 ERCPs (1–13), CT scans (in 73% of patients), and tissue sampling (in 61%). Complications occurred in 3 patients, including 2 cases of mild pancreatitis and 1 perforation that was managed nonoperatively.

Although the presence of biliary stones was known in advance of the procedure in only 5 patients, they were identified in 23 of 41 (56%), including 7 of 23 (30%) by cholangioscopy alone. Stone clearance was accomplished in 10 patients, partial clearance in 7, and it was not attempted in 6. Of 9 patients treated by cholangioscopically directed electrohydraulic or mechanical (n = 3) lithotripsy, 7 achieved complete clearance. Of 8 patients treated by conventional ERCP methods, only 3 achieved complete clearance. Partial or complete stone clearance, with or without stenting or dilation maneuvers, yielded clinical improvement in 77% of patients.

In the same series, 33 of 41 patients with PSC underwent biopsy of lesions noted at cholangioscopy, and 11 returned for repeated biopsy sessions. Indications for biopsy were the same as those used in patients without PSC, namely presence of intraductal masses, infiltrative or ulcerated strictures, and papillary or villous mucosal projections.[8] Sampling of visually identified lesions was performed in all instances; however, in 8 of 44 sessions, sampling could be accomplished only via fluoroscopic guidance after cholangioscopic identification of the area of concern, because of angulation and inability to pass the cholangioscopic forceps to the lesion. In one-quarter of procedures, the stricture of interest could not be traversed with the cholangioscope; however, visually or fluoroscopically directed samples could still be obtained in 9 of 14 (68%) such cases. Samples were obtained from intrahepatic lesions in 15 procedures, extrahepatic lesions in 22, and both locations in 7. Histology findings were positive for cholangiocarcinoma in 1 patient, suspicious or negative in 31, and inadequate in 1. Brush cytology results were suspicious in 2 patients, inadequate in 3, and negative or atypical in 13. Seventeen-month follow-up (range, 1–56 mo) in 40 patients noted carcinoma in only 2, both of whom had transhepatic tubes in place and were examined via percutaneous cholangioscopy; only 1 of the 2 had biopsies deemed suspicious. The investigators emphasized that the visual examination of strictures was often misleading and did not reliably differentiate malignant from benign disease. They advised directed sampling of all epithelial ulcers or masslike projections.

Tischendorf and colleagues[9] from Hanover, Germany, investigated the diagnostic value of visual inspection during cholangioscopy for differentiating benign from malignant biliary strictures during ERCP in patients with PSC. Fifty-three patients were evaluated for PSC with dominant strictures during a 5-year period, ending in 2002. ERCP, sphincterotomy, stricture dilation (4–8 mm), and cholangioscopy were performed in the usual fashion following prophylactic antibiotics. Cholangiography was used to characterize the strictures as benign to malignant on a 4-point scale, based on the radiographic assessment of their length (< 1 cm interpreted as benign, >1 cm interpreted as malignant) and configuration (regular margin vs irregular margin). Cholangioscopy was able to traverse the dominant lesions in all patients using a 9F (2.97 mm) instrument (Almikro Ltd, Bad Krozingen, Germany). Strictures were classified as suspicious for malignancy if irregular ulceration or polypoid or villous mass features were seen. At each procedure, cholangioscopy was followed by stricture sampling via forceps biopsy and/or cytology brushing. The sampling technique was not explicitly described, but it seems as if it was via fluoroscopic guidance. There were no complications attributable to the cholangioscopic examinations.

Twelve of 53 patients (23%) were found to have cholangiocarcinoma. Six patients required more than 1 ERCP with tissue sampling to reach a diagnosis (mean, 2.6 procedures; range, 1–4). Brush cytology results eventually returned positive in 4 of 6 patients, and biopsy results were positive in 10 of 10 cases.

Carefully scored cholangiography alone correctly identified cancer in 8 of 12 cases (sensitivity 66%) and benign lesions in 21 of 41 cases (specificity 51%). In contrast, the cholangioscopic visual examination correctly identified 11 of 12 cancers (92% sensitive) and 38 of 41 benign lesions (93% specific), yielding significantly higher accuracy and positive and negative predictive values (**Table 1**). Nine of 12 cancers exhibited polypoid or villous changes, 2 were ulcerated, and 1 with erosive changes was interpreted as benign. Benign strictures varied from smooth and bland scarring to erythematous and even ulcerated lesions. Three ulcerated lesions were incorrectly interpreted as malignant. This study did not address the potential additional benefits of resources conserved or investigations avoided, by use of visually directed biopsy at the time of cholangioscopy.

The study by Tischendorf and colleagues[9] provides the most descriptive data, to date, on the cholangioscopic findings of cancer in PSC. However, not all studies have noted such visually obvious and easily differentiated features in cholangiocarcinoma complicating PSC, and the specificity of polypoid or villous lesions has been questioned. Recall that Awadallah and colleagues[7] noted lesions in PSC to be very nonspecific and advised obtaining visually directed biopsies whenever possible. Similarly, Dechene and colleagues[10] failed to identify any cancers among 17 patients with PSC, despite cholangioscopic visualization of predefined stigmata of malignancy in 11, including the presence of benign polypoid masses in 4 and villous protrusions in 5. None had ulceration or tortuous "tumor vessels."

The SpyGlass Direct Visualization System (Boston Scientific, Natick, MA, USA) has also been used for evaluation of indeterminate biliary strictures in patients with PSC.[11] In a recently closed multicenter study, evaluation of patients with PSC constituted about 10% of all procedures and about 14% of indeterminate stricture cases. Separate data are not yet available for assessment of indeterminate strictures in patients with PSC versus patients who do not have PSC. Overall, the study confirms the utility

Table 1
Results for interpretation of cholangiocarcinoma in patients with PSC, based on carefully scored cholangiographic images and direct visual examination by cholangioscopy (N = 53)

	ERC			Cholangioscopy			P
	N	%	CI (%)	N	%	CI (%)	
Sensitivity	8/12	66	35 (90)	11/12	92	62 (99.8)	0.25
Specificity	21/41	51	35 (67)	38/41	93	80 (98)	< 0.001
Accuracy	29/53	55	40 (68)	49/53	93	82 (98)	< 0.001
PPV	8/28	29	13 (49)	11/14	79	49 (95)	< 0.001
NPV	21/25	84	64 (95)	38/39	97	87 (99.9)	< 0.025

Abbreviations: CI, 95% confidence interval; ERC, endoscopic retrograde cholangiography; N, number of patients; NPV, negative predictive value; PPV, positive predictive value.

Data from Tischendorf JJW, Kruger M, Trautwein C, et al.Cholangioscopic characterization of dominant bile duct stenoses in patients with primary sclerosing cholangitis. Endoscopy 2006;38:665–9.

of direct visualization for tissue acquisition during assessment of indeterminate strictures. These results are reviewed elsewhere in this issue.

Advanced imaging capabilities such as NBI and chromoendoscopy have been described as useful in the diagnosis of de novo cholangiocarcinoma without PSC.[12] Additional studies are currently under way at the author's institution to assess the potential value of digital video cholangioscopy coupled with NBI for assessment of dominant lesions in PSC.

CHOLANGIOSCOPY IN PATIENTS AFTER LIVER TRANSPLANTATION

Cholangioscopy can be used in the liver transplant patient for the same spectrum of issues as in the nontransplant patient, for example, visual characterization of radiographic abnormalities, visual inspection and directed sampling of indeterminate strictures, visually directed lithotripsy using probe-delivered electrohydraulic or laser energy, and visually guided passage of wires or other devices into specific ducts. Nevertheless, few transplant-specific reports have been published.

Within a larger review of cholangioscopic experience, Siddique and colleagues[13] described 20 procedures in orthotopic liver transplant (OLT) patients. Unexpected fungal infection was apparently identified in the index patient of this group, prompting protocolized cholangioscopy for evaluation of 14 patients with anastomotic strictures and 6 with elevated liver function tests. Overall, in 5 of 20 patients, the donor bile-duct mucosa exhibited a dull grayish appearance, suggesting possible ischemia. Among those with anastomotic strictures, 8 had ulceration and severe inflammatory changes in the donor bile ducts, 4 had mild inflammatory changes, and 2 had cicatricial strictures. Brush sampling identified cytomegalovirus inclusions in 2 patients and fungal elements in 1, all among the group with severe inflammatory changes. Findings among the 6 OLT patients with elevated liver enzyme levels included 2 normal studies and individual cases of intrahepatic stone, intraductal clot, retained suture with adherent stone debris, and stricture requiring cholangioscopic wire guidance for drainage.

Perhaps the most unique biliary challenges in the transplantation setting are those related to duct ischemia and the subsequent intraductal cast syndrome or widespread strictures in the transplanted biliary tree. Ischemic biliary strictures are the most frequent nonanastomotic biliary complication following transplantation, occurring in 2% to 19% of patients.[14] One recent report described use of cholangioscopy with methylene blue chromoendoscopy to characterize differential uptake of the vital stain between areas of necrosis and viable perfused mucosa. Subtle abnormalities of early mucosal ischemia and the extent of involvement were more readily evident than by cholangiography alone.[15] The authors proposed potential further roles for cholangioscopy of ischemic ducts. Intuitively, it might be anticipated that NBI would provide similar delineation of ischemic mucosa and cholangioscopically directed probes might allow functional characterization of healthy, ischemic, and at-risk biliary mucosa.

Several additional case reports also suggest potential utility for cholangioscopy in OLT patients. They include use of the SpyGlass Direct Visualization System for localization and wire passage through a tight anastomotic stricture that could not be traversed by other means[16] and use of percutaneous cholangioscopy for management of a completely closed choledocho-jejunal anastomosis that would not allow passage of contrast.[17] Much like the rendezvous techniques that use simultaneous antegrade-retrograde access to tunnel through totally closed esophageal strictures,[18] in this case, the antegrade cholangioscope was passed via percutaneous access to the intrahepatic side of the completely strictured anastomosis and a double balloon enteroscope was passed to the distal jejunal side. Light transmission was readily seen from each side, providing visual guidance for wire puncture, dilation, and stenting from above. We recently employed cholangioscopy during serial procedures to effect complete electrohydraulic lithotripsy and clearance of a large (2 cm) symptomatic stone contained within an intrahepatic gallbladder that was implanted together with the surrounding liver.

CHOLANGIOSCOPY FOR SELECTIVE DUCT ACCESS

The use of cholangioscopic guidance to enable access to specific ducts or segments of the biliary tree is often mentioned as an addendum to the more common stricture- and stone-oriented applications of cholangioscopy.[19] The technique usually uses standard 450-cm-length, 0.035-in guidewires to facilitate removal of the cholangioscope and over-the-wire exchange to other dilating, grasping, or stenting devices. This requires significant caution to avoid loss of access that has been achieved. Angled, slippery wires facilitate access efforts, even with steerable cholangioscope designs. Short, slippery wires can be used if directed access is intended only for cholangioscopically guided therapy or sampling, as in intrahepatic sampling or stone therapy.

Selected duct access remains an uncommon niche indication for cholangioscopy because of the usual success with currently used devices, the cumbersome nature of dedicated reusable cholangioscopes, and the significant expense of the partially disposable SpyGlass Direct Visualization System. In the multicenter study of that system, cholangioscopy was used to facilitate directed wire access in only 5 out of 296 cases.[20] In the author's experience, the technique is infrequently needed when the technical challenge involves traversing a single tight stricture that can be radiographically defined with contrast and approached with common balloons and guidewires. Cholangioscopic guidance may prove useful in several settings, however. Examples include the challenges when accessing a stricture that is just beyond an acute angulation or a duct that enters a confluence at an acute angle; when the duct of interest is one among many entering a confluence, yet is visually distinct (by blood or pus); or when a small tortuous duct joins a large-caliber system (such as the cystic-common hepatic duct junction). Cholangioscopy or pancreatoscopy can also be used, as a last resort, to enable wire passage into proximally migrated plastic stents, which can then be removed by wire-guided snare or balloon retrieval.

Conceptually, cholangioscopy for directed wire access is entirely analogous to visually directed biopsy, injection, lithotripsy, basket capture, or any other focal application of endoscopic devices or therapies. All are more accurately and efficiently deployed under direct visual guidance than via 2-dimensional fluoroscopic guidance. Imagine the use of fluoroscopy to guide thermal therapy of a vascular malformation or to enable snaring a pedunculated polyp in the colon! The analogy helps visualize the potential utility of cholangioscopy for various interventions. The barriers are not insignificant; they include the need for technical development of smaller devices and potential limitations in the endoscopists' time, talent, and treasure (eg, financial constraints).

SUMMARY

With the recent improvements in mini-scope technology, including video systems, NBI capability, and the development of a reliable single-operator system, cholangioscopy is gaining renewed interest and gradually expanded use. Challenging clinical dilemmas that may benefit from its application include early diagnosis of cholangiocarcinoma in the setting of PSC, early identification of biliary infection or ischemia following OLT, and achieving selective duct access with wires and other devices during therapeutic ERCP.

REFERENCES

1. Maggs J, Chapman R. An update on primary sclerosing cholangitis. Curr Opin Gastroenterol 2008;24:377–83.
2. Fevery J, Verslype C, Lai G, et al. Incidence, diagnosis, and therapy of cholangio-carcinoma in patients with primary sclerosing cholangitis. Dig Dis Sci 2007;52:3123–35.
3. Heimbach J. Successful liver transplantation for hilar cholangiocarcinoma. Curr Opin Gastroenterol 2008;24:384–8.
4. Morena Luna LE, Gores GJ. Advances in the diagnosis of cholangiocarcinoma in patients with primary sclerosing cholangitis. Liver Transpl 2006;12:S15–9.
5. Berquist A, Glaumann H, Persson B, et al. Risk factors and clinical presentation of hepatobiliary carcinoma in patients with primary sclerosing cholangitis: a case-control study. Hepatology 1998;27:311–6.
6. DeHaan RD, Kipp R, Smyrk TC, et al. An assessment of chromosomal alterations detected by fluorescence in situ hybridization and p16 expression in sporadic and primary sclerosing cholangitis associated cholangiocarcinomas. Hum Pathol 2007;38:491–9.
7. Awadallah NS, Chen YK, Piraka C, et al. Is there a role for cholangioscopy in patients with primary sclerosing cholangitis? Am J Gastroenterol 2006;101:284–91.
8. Seo DW, Lee SK, Yoo KS, et al. Cholangioscopic findings in bile duct tumors. Gastrointest Endosc 2000;52:630–4.
9. Tischendorf JJW, Kruger M, Trautwein C, et al. Cholangioscopic characterization of dominant bile duct stenoses in patients with primary sclerosing cholangitis. Endoscopy 2006;38:665–9.
10. Dechene A, Hilgard PA, Fouly AE, et al. It looks like cholangiocarcinoma – but is it? cholangioscopy using a cholangioscopy system for diagnosis of cholangiocar-cinoma in patients with primary sclerosing cholangitis [abstract]. Gastrointest Endosc 2009;69:AB116.
11. Pleskow D, Parsi MA, Chen YK, et al. Biopsy of indeterminate biliary strictures - does direct visualization help? - A multicenter experience [abstract]. Gastrointest Endosc 2008;67(5):AB103.
12. Itoi T, Sofuni A, Itokawa F, et al. Peroral cholangioscopic diagnosis of biliary-tract diseases by using narrow-band imaging. Gastrointest Endosc 2007;66:730–6.
13. Siddique I, Galati J, Ankoma-Sey V, et al. The role of choledochoscopy in the diagnosis and management of biliary tract diseases. Gastrointest Endosc 1999;50:67–73.
14. Bandsaeter B, Schrumpf E, Clausen OP, et al. Recurrent sclerosing cholangitis or ischemic bile duct lesions – a diagnostic challenge. Liver Transpl 2004;10:1073–4.
15. Hoffman A, Kiesslich R, Moench C, et al. Methylene blue-aided cholangioscopy unravels the endoscopic features of ischemic-type biliary lesions after liver trans-plantation. Gastrointest Endosc 2007;66:1052–8.
16. Wright H, Sharma S, Gurakar A, et al. Management of biliary stricture guided by the spyglass direct visualization system in a liver transplant recipient: an innova-tive approach. Gastrointest Endosc 2008;67:1201–3.

17. Tsukui D, Yano T, Nakazawa K, et al. Rendezvous technique combining double-balloon endoscopy with percutaneous cholangioscopy is useful for the treatment of biliary anastomotic obstruction after liver transplantation. Gastrointest Endosc 2008;68:1013–5.
18. Maple JT, Petersen BT, Baron TH, et al. Endoscopic management of radiation-induced complete upper esophageal obstruction with an antegrade-retrograde rendezvous technique. Gastrointest Endosc 2006;64:822–8.
19. Shah RJ, Adler DG, Conway JD, et al. ASGE technology status evaluation report: cholangioscopy. Gastrointest Endosc 2008;69(3):411–21.
20. Chen Y, Parsi MA, Binmoller KF, et al. Peroral Cholangioscopy (POC) using a disposable steerable single operator catheter for biliary stone therapy and assessment of indeterminate strictures: a multi-center experience using SPYGLASS [abstract]. Gastrointest Endosc 2009;69(5):AB264–5.

Choledochoscopy-Assisted Intraductal Shock Wave Lithotripsy

Jason Bratcher, MD[a], Franklin Kasmin, MD[b],*

KEYWORDS

- Lithotripsy • Choledocholithiasis • Choledochoscopy
- Electrohydraulic • Laser • ERCP

Cholelithiasis is an increasingly prevalent disorder in the United States, affecting more than 6 million men and 14 million women annually.[1] Of this population, choledocholithiasis occurs in up to 20%, and is a common indication for referral to a specialist in biliary endoscopy.[2] In more than 90% of these cases, endoscopic retrograde cholangiopancreatography (ERCP) with sphincterotomy and stone extraction are successful therapeutic options for clearance of the bile duct with the use of a stone retrieval balloon or basket. Large or impacted stones may require fragmentation for removal, which can be accomplished in most cases with mechanical lithotripsy.[3–5] In a small percentage of patients with biliary stones, however, these traditional techniques fail, and advanced techniques for fragmentation must be used. Reasons for failure are usually due to the size of the stone, with stones larger than 1.5 to 2 cm causing the most difficulty with traditional extraction methods, or the presence of biliary strictures that increase the complexity of stone removal.[6,7]

Intraductal shock wave lithotripsy offers the endoscopist a therapeutic option that may be effective despite the difficulties of a large, impacted stone that cannot be captured by a basket, or a stricture that prohibits delivery of a stone beyond it. By employing a technology deliverable via a thin fiber, lithotripsy of even the most complicated stones can be achieved. Although fluoroscopically guided intraductal shock wave lithotripsy techniques have been developed, to date most procedures have been performed with the guidance of a choledochoscope placed through a standard or oversized side-viewing endoscope. Thus, as a result of the cost of materials and time required for these procedures, they are generally withheld unless standard techniques have failed.

[a] Division of Gastroenterology, Beth Israel Medical Center, 10 Nathan Perlman Place, First Avenue at 16th Street, New York, NY 10003, USA
[b] Division of Gastroenterology, The Pancreas and Biliary Center, St Vincent's Hospital, 170 W 12th Street, New York, NY 10011, USA
* Corresponding author.
E-mail address: FKNY@aol.com (F. Kasmin).

Gastrointest Endoscopy Clin N Am 19 (2009) 587–595
doi:10.1016/j.giec.2009.07.004
1052-5157/09/$ – see front matter © 2009 Published by Elsevier Inc.

giendo.theclinics.com

ELECTROHYDRAULIC LITHOTRIPSY

Originally developed by the Soviet Union as an industrial tool for breaking large rocks, electrohydraulic lithotripsy (EHL) has become a useful tool in the management of in vivo stone disease. The first reported human use was in the treatment of urolithiasis in 1970[8] and in 1975, the first use for treatment of retained bile duct stones was described by Burhenne, using access to the bile duct via a percutaneous biliary tube.[9] Shortly thereafter, Koch and colleagues described the endoscopic use of the new technique using a lithotripsy probe and basket for biliary stone disease.[10] Since this breakthrough, multiple studies have proven this method as an effective modality for treating difficult biliary stones in a purely endoscopic fashion.

EHL employs a 1.9F fiber that passes through a catheter or choledochoscope channel to the lumen of the bile duct. The duct also must contain a catheter or other mode of irrigation, as EHL requires copious irrigation, and is used with normal saline to allow for water vaporization and transmission of the shock waves.[11] The fiber is connected externally to an electric generator (**Fig. 1**) that produces up to 30 electrical impulses per second, which are transmitted to the noninsulated double-electrode tip of the fiber in the duct lumen. With each discharge of electrical current, a small amount of water at the tip of the probe is vaporized, and the change in state from water to gas produces a release of energy that is transmitted through the water in a waveform. This energy is transmitted to the stone if the fiber tip is held close to the stone, and fragmentation of the stone can occur. The procedure is repeated until the stone is broken into pieces that can be removed by basket or balloon extraction (**Fig. 2**).

Early use of EHL depended on fluoroscopic guidance to position the probe against the stone. The first report described the passage of the probe through the catheter of a stone basket, such that the stone would be held in place by the basket and the probe would be directed against the stone as it emerged form the basket lumen. Siegel and colleagues[12] described the passage of the EHL fiber through the large-diameter lumen of a specially designed balloon extraction catheter. With the balloon inflated below the stone, the tip of the catheter was held centrally within the duct, such that as the fiber emerged from the catheter, it was located centrally and near the stone. Each of these techniques had a host of technical hurdles to overcome. Also, 2-dimensional

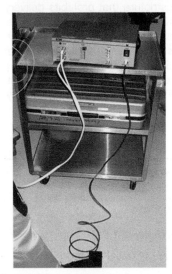

Fig. 1. ACMI generator for electrohydraulic lithotripsy.

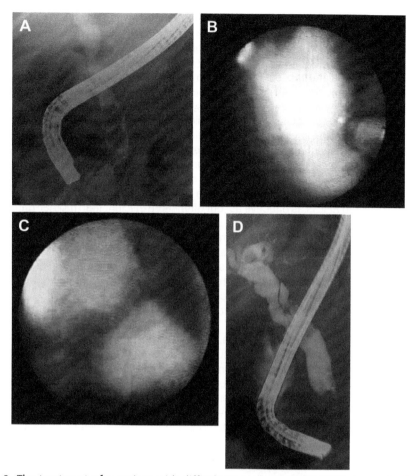

Fig. 2. The treatment of a patient with difficult stones by EHL. (*A*) ERCP demonstrating 2 large impacted stones. (*B*) EHL probe against stone, ready for lithotripsy, as seen during choledochoscopy. (*C*) Stone fragments after EHL. (*D*) Clearance of stones.

fluoroscopic guidance could not ensure that the EHL probe tip was not against or near the duct wall, and ductal injury at times ensued.

To avoid the shortcomings of the fluoro-guided techniques of EHL, direct cholangio-scopy was used to guide EHL. The initial choledochoscopes were 4.5-mm instruments that required a 5.4-mm channel side-view endoscope to pass them up the duct. This "mother-daughter" system had only one channel, measuring 1.6 mm, and no separate water irrigation system. However, with the use of a side-arm adapter, one could lavage the duct around the indwelling probe, and reasonably efficient EHL was possible under direct vision. The instrument could be manipulated into the intrahepatic system with regularity, and could be advanced over a wire beyond a stricture following dila-tion. Once the stone was visualized and successfully lithotripted, the mother-daughter system was removed and a standard side-view endoscope was passed; fragments were treated with standard endoscopic techniques, or failures were treated with the placement of an indwelling stent. An advance occurred in the late 1990s with the development of a "baby" choledochoscope that could be passed through the 4.2-mm channel of a standard large-channel duodenoscope. The 1.2-mm channel of the daughter scope allows less room for the passage of water around the indwelling EHL probe, and so a high pressure delivery system—usually a liter of saline compressed by a blood pressure cuff—is connected to the side-arm adaptor at the baby scope's channel. Removal of the baby scope following the completion of EHL allowed the immediate application of therapy, as the standard duodenoscope was already in position. Nonetheless, both of these systems were generally 2-operator systems and EHL typically was an ordeal lasting 1 to 2 hours.

The advent of the "Spyglass" system has simplified EHL (**Fig. 3**). As the Spy system catheter is a disposable dual-plane deflection tool with a dedicated large-caliber probe insertion channel and a separate water irrigation port, each of the processes of EHL, namely access, probe, passage, and lavage, is improved. Like the baby scope, Spy-assisted EHL is done through a standard large-channel duodenoscope, though the whole system is designed to be controlled by one operator. It is likely that Spy-assisted EHL is as effective as, but often more efficient than mother-daughter or mother-baby assisted procedures.

Regardless of the techniques used, multiple applications may be necessary in the same setting, and debris and fragments that obscure direct visualization often must be cleared with irrigation or endoscopic suction. Much of the manipulation of the cholangioscope is done by manipulation of the duodenoscope shaft and tip controls, and most of the duct luminal suctioning is accomplished by the duodenoscope's suction of the duodenum, which encourages passage of debris and irrigated water out through the sphincterotomy site.

Success rates using EHL are variable, and depend on whether other methods are used concurrently. Using EHL alone, a success rate of 40% to 80% can be expected. Most studies use a combination of techniques, such as mechanical lithotripsy, extracorporeal shock wave lithotripsy (ESWL), or laser lithotripsy, along with EHL. The addition of multiple treatment modalities increases the overall success rate to more than 90%.[13–18] The largest study of EHL reviewed a 12-year experience covering 93 patients with failed stone extraction attempts due to large stones or difficult ductal

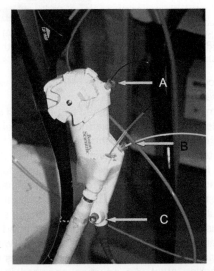

Fig. 3. The Boston Scientific "Spyglass" system loaded onto a standard duodenoscope. A: 1.9F lithotripsy electrode taped to "Spy" handle and passed into biopsy channel. B: Spyglass visualization fiber in dedicated channel. C: dedicated irrigation port.

anatomy. At least some stone fragmentation was possible in 89 of the 93 patients, and 24% required multiple EHL sessions. A final stone clearance of 90% was achieved.[18] Riemann's group compared EHL with ESWL in a randomized study of 35 patients with difficult stones. The ESWL group had fragmentation in 15 of 18 patients (83%), and there was successful fragmentation in 13 of 17 patients (76%) of the EHL patients. Both techniques typically required multiple sessions, and the stone clearance rate (about 70%) was similar in both groups.[19]

In addition to the usual complications that arise from the initial ERCP with sphincter-otomy, adverse events can happen with EHL, but are rare. Bile duct injury leading to bleeding or perforation can occur if the probe is not placed in direct contact with the stone or if direct visualization is compromised.[20]

LASER LITHOTRIPSY

Laser (Light Amplification of Stimulated Emission of Radiation) was first developed in the 1960s as a method to create a focused beam of energy for a variety of uses, which quickly led to investigations of therapeutic uses in medical applications.[21,22] Gastro-enterology has benefited from the technology in many different scenarios, ranging from tissue ablation in patients with cancer to hemostasis of bleeding angiodyspla-sias.[23] Due to the ability to produce a high-power shock wave, fragmentation of stone disease was a natural fit for this new therapeutic modality. In the early 1980s, Japa-nese investigators used laser lithotripsy in the treatment of common bile duct stones via a percutaneous approach with a choledochoscope.[24,25] The type of laser used consisted of a continuous wave Neodynium:YAG laser using a quartz fiber passed through a basket containing the stone. This laser converts light into thermal energy, and was demonstrated to cause melting of or drilling into stones rather than the frag-mentation necessary for clearance from the bile duct. Because the laser is activated for several seconds at a time, the continuous energy generated increases the risk of bile duct injury and fragments stones into large pieces, making endoscopic removal difficult. Furthermore, this laser was found to be useful only for bilirubin stones and did not work for cholesterol stones.[25]

Subsequent studies found that by changing to a rapid pulse laser rather than a continuous wave laser, fragmentation could be achieved by generating an enormous amount of energy (in the gigawatt range) for only fractions of a second at a time, thus reducing the risk of thermal injury to the bile duct.[26,27] The first experiments using this technique were used for the treatment of urolithiasis, and employed flashlamp-pulsed Nd:YAG lasers. By converting light into thermal energy for only nanoseconds at a time, stone fragmentation was successful and heat generation was well below the threshold for creating serious tissue trauma.[27] Although the amount of generated heat was low, the theoretical risk of thermal injury remained, and the search for a more effective and safe alternative continued.

The development of the pulsed-dye laser allowed for the use of shock waves rather than thermal energy to fragment stones. The concept involves the laser-generated formation of plasma at the surface of the stone. A bubble then develops, which expands and then collapses, creating an acoustic shock wave with an intense shearing force to the liquid at the surface of the stone (**Fig. 4**). The force generated by the acoustic wave, rather than thermal energy, allows for the creation of large amounts of energy without the damaging effects to the biliary epithelium.[28] The first human experiments using this technology via an endoscopic approach were per-formed by Ell and colleagues in 1988.[29] Nine patients were enrolled in the study, 8 of whom achieved the end point of gallstone fragmentation. However, in 2 of these

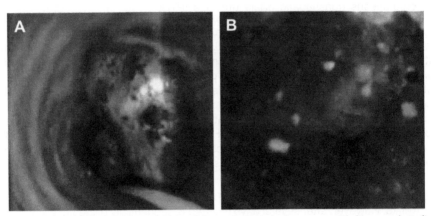

Fig. 4. Laser lithotripsy. (*A*) Stone as viewed through choledochoscope, with fiber ready to fire. (*B*) Fragmentation during firing of the laser. (*Courtesy of* Juergen Hochberger, MD, PhD.)

patients the fragments were too large to be removed endoscopically, requiring surgery in one and internal biliary drainage in the other, but no complications occurred in this study. Cotton and colleagues subsequently studied 25 patients with difficult-to-treat common bile duct stones using pulsed-dye laser lithotripsy.[30] In 19 patients, an endoscopic approach was used with a mother-baby duodenoscope, and in 6, a transcutaneous approach was used through existing biliary drains. The overall success rate was 80%, with 20 patients achieving duct clearance that required multiple sessions in 8 cases. No major complications were noted, but one patient developed self-limited bile duct bleeding after laser therapy. Ponchon and colleagues reported that direct visualization is crucial to treatment with laser lithotripsy.[31] In their series, the bile duct was able to be completely cleared in all patients who underwent direct visualization (11 of 25 patients) versus only 5 of 14 cases under fluoroscopic control. This finding demonstrates the necessity of proper positioning, and visually ensuring the laser probe is in direct contact with stone for maximal benefit.

Newer laser technologies of interest include the Holmium:YAG laser and the systems that provide automated tissue recognition. The Holmium:YAG system was initially developed in the late 1990s for ureteral stone disease, and was soon thereafter utilized in the biliary tract. Direct visualization is necessary to prevent tissue damage and ensure efficacy, so the probe is placed through percutaneous or endoscopically placed choledochoscopes. A variety of laser types have since been developed, but the most commonly used devices today are the coumarin dye laser and the rhodamine 6G dye laser.[30,32] Tissue recognition systems have also been developed, such as the Lithognost laser, which have increased the ability to differentiate biliary epithelium from stones during the application of the energy beam, further reducing the risk of bile duct damage.[33] This type of laser analyzes back-scattered light, causing an interruption in signal when the reflected light indicates that tissue has been encountered. The net effect is a reduction of over 95% in the total transmitted laser energy, thus reducing potential trauma. Neuhaus and colleagues demonstrated the efficacy of this system by completely clearing the common bile duct in 37 of 38 patients with stones refractory to traditional therapy, 5 of whom were under fluoroscopic guidance alone.[34]

Laser lithotripsy is similar to EHL in that both transcutaneous and endoscopic approaches can be successfully used. The transhepatic method involves the insertion of the laser probe via a choledochoscope into a preexisting precutaneous biliary tract. The purely endoscopic approach uses mother-baby choledochoscope technology. Using the latter technique, a 4-mm diameter choledochoscope is passed under direct vision into the bile duct. The laser probe, consisting of a highly flexible 0.2-mm quartz fiber, is positioned into direct contact with the stone. Stabilization of the probe can be accomplished with the use of balloon catheters, basket catheters, or sleeved catheters, which help to ensure proper contact between the laser probe and the stone.[30,34] Laser energy is transmitted at 504 nm through a Candela flashlamp excited dye laser.

Efficacy of laser lithotripsy ranges from 80% to more than 90% in most studies, and most patients remained stone-free during follow-up evaluation.[33,35,36] The presence of biliary strictures and low body mass index were significant risk factors for stone recurrence, which was encountered in 15% of patients in one study.[37]

SUMMARY

Choledocholithiasis is a common medical problem that can usually be managed by ERCP with sphincterotomy and stone extraction in the vast majority of cases. Large stones or the presence of biliary strictures occasionally prevent the clearance of the bile duct, and alternative methods can be used to preclude surgical intervention. Intraductal treatment of biliary stones using electrohydraulic or laser lithotripsy is effective in up to 90% of cases that have failed traditional endoscopic removal, and have been shown to be safe when performed by skilled biliary endoscopists. This technology is not universally available, however, and is usually performed in tertiary referral centers by experts in biliary endoscopy.

REFERENCES

1. Everhart JE, Khare M, Hill M, et al. Prevalence and ethnic differences in gallbladder disease in the United States. Gastroenterology 1999;117(3):632–9.
2. Hermann RE. The spectrum of biliary stone disease. Am J Surg 1989;158(3): 171–3.
3. Siegel JH. Endoscopic papillotomy: sphincterotomy or sphincteroplasty. Am J Gastroenterol 1979;72:511–6.
4. Cotton PG. Endoscopic management of bile duct stones (apples and oranges). Gut 1984;25:587–97.
5. Sivak MV. Endoscopic management of bile duct stones. Am J Surg 1989;158: 228–40.
6. Classen M, Hagenmuller F, Knyrim K, et al. Giant bile duct stones—nonsurgical treatment. Endoscopy 1988;20:21–6.
7. Katon RM. The giant common duct stone: still a hard nut to crack. Gastrointest Endosc 1988;34:281–2.
8. Reuter HJ. Electrical lithotripsy. A new method for treating calculi of the bladder and ureter. J Urol Nephrol (Paris) 1971;77(Suppl):551–3.
9. Burhenne HJ. Electrohydrolytic fragmentation of retained common duct stones. Radiology 1975;117(3 Pt 1):721–3.
10. Koch H, Stolte M, Walz V. Endoscopic lithotripsy in the common bile duct. Endoscopy 1977;9(2):95–8.
11. Baron T, Kozareck R, Carr-Locke D. ERCP. Philadelphia: Saunders; 2008. p. 127.
12. Siegel JH, Ben-Zvi JS, Pullano WE. Endoscopic electrohydraulic lithotripsy. Gastrointest Endosc 1990;36(2):134–6.

13. Binmoeller KF, Bruckner M, Thonke F, et al. Treatment of difficult bile duct stones using mechanical, electrohydraulic and extracorporeal shock wave lithotripsy. Endoscopy 1993;25(3):201–6.

14. Adamek HE, Schneider AR, Adamek MU, et al. Treatment of difficult intrahepatic stones by using extracorporeal and intracorporeal lithotripsy techniques: 10 years' experience in 55 patients. Scand J Gastroenterol 1999;34(11): 1157–61.

15. Adamek HE, Maier M, Jakobs R, et al. Management of retained bile duct stones: a prospective open trial comparing extracorporeal and intracorporeal lithotripsy. Gastrointest Endosc 1996;44(1):40–7.

16. Hui CK, Lai KC, Ng M, et al. Retained common bile duct stones: a comparison between biliary stenting and complete clearance of stones by electrohydraulic lithotripsy. Aliment Pharmacol Ther 2003;17(2):289–96.

17. Moon JH, Cha SW, Ryu CB, et al. Endoscopic treatment of retained bile-duct stones by using a balloon catheter for electrohydraulic lithotripsy without cholangioscopy. Gastrointest Endosc 2004;60(4):562–6.

18. Arya N, Nelles SE, Haber GB, et al. Electrohydraulic lithotripsy in 111 patients: a safe and effective therapy for difficult bile duct stones. Am J Gastroenterol 2004;99(12):2330–4.

19. Adamek HE, Buttmann A, Wessbecher R, et al. Clinical comparison of extracorporeal piezoelectric lithotripsy (EPL) and intracorporeal electrohydraulic lithotripsy (EHL) in difficult bile duct stones. A prospective randomized trial. Dig Dis Sci 1995;40(6):1185–92.

20. Harrison J, Morris DL, Haynes J, et al. Electrohydraulic lithotripsy of gallstones-in vitro and animal studies. Gut 1987;28:267–71.

21. Gould R. Gordon. "The LASER, Light Amplification by Stimulated Emission of Radiation". The Ann Arbor Conference on Optical Pumping. University of Michigan, 15 June through 18 June 1959:128.

22. Sliney DH, Trokel SL. Medical lasers and their safe use. New York: Springer Verlag; 1993.

23. Zopf T, Riemann JF. The change in laser usage in gastroenterology—the status in 1997. Z Gastroenterol 1997;35(11):987–97.

24. Orii K, Nakahara A, Takase Y, et al. Choledocholithotomy by YAG laser with a choledochofiberscope; case reports of two patients. Surgery 1981;90:120–2.

25. Orii K, Ozaki A, Takase Y, et al. Lithotomy of intrahepatic and choledochal stones with YAG-laser. Surg Gynecol Obstet 1983;156:485.

26. Ell C, Wondrazxek F, Frank F, et al. Laser-induced shockwave lithotripsy of gallstones. Endoscopy 1986;18:95–6.

27. Ell C, Hockberger J, Muller D, et al. Laser lithotripsy of gallstone by means of a pulsed Neodynium-Yag laser—in vitro and animal experiments. Endoscopy 1986;18:92–4.

28. Teng P, Nishioka NS, Farinelli WA, et al. Microsecond-long flash photography of laser-induced ablation of biliary and urinary calculi. Lasers Surg Med 1987;7: 394–7.

29. Ell C, Lux G, Hochberger J, et al. Laser lithotripsy of common bile duct stones. Gut 1988;29:746–51.

30. Cotton PB, Kozarek RA, Schapiro RH, et al. Endoscopic laser lithotripsy of large bile duct stones. Gastroenterology 1990;99(4):1128–33.

31. Ponchon T, Gagnon P, Valette PJ, et al. Pulsed dye laser lithotripsy of bile duct stones. Gastroenterology 1991;100(6):1730–6.

32. Ell C, Hochberger J, May A, et al. Hahn Laser lithotripsy of difficult bile duct stones by means of a rhodamine-6G laser and an integrated automatic stone-tissue detection system. Gastrointest Endosc 1993;39(6):755–62.
33. Neuhaus H, Hoffman W, Gottlieb K, et al. Endoscopic lithotripsy of bile duct stones using a new laser with automatic stone recognition. Gastrointest Endosc 1994;40:708–15.
34. Neuhaus H, Hoffmann W, Zillinger C, et al. Laser lithotripsy of difficult bile duct stones under direct visual control. Gut 1993;34(3):415–21.
35. Hochberger J, Tex S, Maiss J, et al. Management of difficult common bile duct stones. Gastrointest Endosc Clin N Am 2003;13(4):623–34.
36. Jakobs R, Maier M, Kohler B, et al. Peroral laser lithotripsy of difficult intrahepatic and extrahepatic bile duct stones: laser effectiveness using an automatic stone-tissue discrimination system. Am J Gastroenterol 1996;91(3):468–73.
37. Jakobs R, Hartmann D, Kudis V, et al. Risk factors for symptomatic stone recurrence after transpapillary laser lithotripsy for difficult bile duct stones using a laser with a stone recognition system. Eur J Gastroenterol Hepatol 2006;18(5):469–73.

Endoscopic Tumor Treatment in the Bile Duct

Juergen Hochberger, MD, PhD*, Giovanni d'Addazio, MD

KEYWORDS

- Bile duct neoplasms • Cholangiopancreatography
- Endoscopy • Digestive system • Cholangiocarcinoma
- Humans • Bile ducts/pathology

Deister[1] reported on the general value of diagnostic intraoperative cholangioscopy using rigid optics as early as 1963. Classen and Ossenberg[2] performed a successful retrograde minicholangioscopy using a fiberoptic catheter for tumor detection in 1977. Japanese hepatobiliary surgeons have reported on the value of preoperative percutaneous transhepatic cholangioscopy since the early 1980s.[3–9] Other than gastroenterologists, specialized surgeons and interventional radiologists have used percutaneous transhepatic access techniques for tumor diagnosis and palliative treatment.[10]

There is little information in the literature on endoscopic tumor treatment in the bile duct with a curative intention. The main reason may be that detection of benign or malignant tumors in the biliary tree is a rare case in the early stage of disease. Surgery has been the gold standard of care whenever patients are in an operable state. In the past, for those patients unfit for surgery, palliative treatment securing biliary drainage by plastic or metal stents was used most often. Local irradiation using iridium-192 was for the specific local treatment of bile duct cancer, mostly, however, with the aim of palliation.[11] Advanced imaging techniques may allow identifying these cases more often in an early stage in the future (eg, by means of magnetic resonance cholangiopancreatography and high-resolution endoscopic ultrasound [EUS], including digital standard scanners acting from the duodenum or stomach and miniprobes inserted directly into the bile duct).[12]

New disposable catheter cholangioscopes and a new technique of inserting 4.7- to 5.8-mm nasal/fine-caliber endoscopes via a guide wire or balloon catheter have facilitated access to the bile duct using a standard endoscope with a high-resolution video chip and 2-mm channel.[13] Furthermore, electronic processing techniques of the

Department of Medicine III–Gastroenterology, Interventional Endoscopy, St. Bernward Academic Teaching Hospital, Treibe Strasse 9, Hildesheim D – 31134, Germany
* Corresponding author.
E-mail addresses: prof.dr.j.hochberger@bernward-khs.de or juehochber@mac.com
(J. Hochberger).

Gastrointest Endoscopy Clin N Am 19 (2009) 597–600
doi:10.1016/j.giec.2009.07.001
1052-5157/09/$ – see front matter © 2009 Elsevier Inc. All rights reserved.

standard image (eg, narrow band imaging) or electronic image enhancement can be used.[14,15] Regarding therapeutic measures, a miniaturization of coagulation probes allows easy application of argon plasma coagulation (APC) via standard nasal endoscopes in the bile duct.[14] Laser lithotripsy fibers and 3- to 5-Fr electrohydraulic lithotripsy probes also can be applied.[16–18] This article reports on the few cases published on and on the authors' own experience with endoscopic retrograde and percutaneous transhepatic cholangioscopic treatment of tumors in the biliary system.

CHOLANGIOSCOPY FOR THE STAGING AND TREATMENT OF BILIARY NEOPLASMS

Brauer and colleagues[14] describe a case of direct peroral cholangioscopy using a high-resolution nasal gastroscope in a patient with intraductal papillary neoplasm and Billroth II resection with a short afferent limb. They applied APC of 15 to 25 W using a side-firing probe to facilitate precise lateral application. Sweeping the bile duct with 1% N-acetylcysteine proved helpful for clearance of the mucinous material from the duct. Narrow band imaging facilitated defining the proximal and distal extension of the tumor and subsequent ablation treatment. Two treatment sessions were performed and a 7-Fr double pigtail stent was left in place after each treatment. Unfortunately the patient died 1 month later from refractory hepatic encephalopathy due to his underlying prior cryptogenic liver cirrhosis.

Jazrawi describes a similar case of biliary papillomatosis in the distal common bile duct treated by intraductal APC in a 37-year-old patient.[19] The patient had previously undergone a hepatico-jejunostomy, because of papillomatosis and secondary detection of lesions in the distal duct. He refused Whipple's resection and received endoscopic retrograde APC treatment using a high power of 50 W at 1 L of gas flow and 1-s pulses. Four months later, a control revealed no residual of the prior lesion.

Photodynamic therapy was successfully applied in 2 studies with 24 and with 4 patients with advanced bile duct cancer using cholangioscopy and EUS as staging modality and treatment control whereas the treatment itself was performed under purely radiologic control using a diffusor catheter over a percutaneous guide wire.[20,21] Maetani and colleagues reported on three patients with occluded metal stents, citing their prior work (published in Japanese) using microwave coagulation. Since 1994, they had used a percutaneous transhepatic access to apply this technique. In the three patients, they were able to introduce the energy source via a transpapillary sleeve.[22]

ENDOSCOPIC MUCOSAL RESECTION (EMR) AND ENDOSCOPIC SUBMUCOSAL DISSECTION (ESD) IN THE BILE DUCT

EMR and ESD in the common bile duct have not been thought possible in the common bile duct. However, in January 2004, an 80-year-old patient was admitted to the authors' hospital because of progressive jaundice. Ultrasound revealed dilated intra- and extrahepatic bile ducts. Endoscopic retrograde cholangiopancreatography showed an unclear mass in the distal common bile duct resembling primarily a 2.5- × 1.5-cm stone. Because the patient was immobile, biopsies were taken and showed a tubulovillous adenoma of the distal common bile duct with mostly low-grade but focally high-grade dysplasia. EUS and CT scan showed the tumor was limited to the distal common bile duct without involvement of the pancreatic duct and limited to the mucosa. The patient refused surgery but agreed to undergo percutaneous transhepatic puncture, tract dilation, and local resection of the mucosal adenoma. After dilation of tract to 20 Fr, a percutaneous transhepatic cholangioscopy using a standard 5.8-mm cholangio/bronchioscope (Fuji EB470T; Fujinon Corp, Saitama, Japan) was performed. A needle catheter was backloaded and a submucosal injection was performed showing a clear lifting of the tumor. An attempt to place a snare around the polyp, involving two-thirds of the circumference, was unsuccessful. An ESD using a standard needle knife was performed and the tumor excised en bloc. Unfortunately the specimen passed rapidly via the papilla and could not be retrieved with the cholangioscope or a peroral gastroscope, as it had already passed the ligament of Treitz. The further course of the patient was uneventful; the patient was discharged 1 week later. To the authors' knowledge, this is the first, and only reported ESD case in the bile duct (submitted for publication).

ACKNOWLEDGMENT

The authors thank Gabor Egervari, MD, for his support in editing the manuscript.

REFERENCES

1. Deister J. [Intraoperative cholangioscopy, an improvement in bile duct diagnosis]. Langenbecks Arch Klin Chir Ver Dtsch Z Chir 1963;303:111–22 [in German].
2. Classen M, Ossenberg FW. [Modern biliary tract diagnosis: endoscopic-retrograde cholangio-pancreaticography and cholangioscopy]. Med Klin 1977;72:684–93.
3. Nimura Y. [Percutaneous transhepatic cholangioscopy: technics and clinical studies]. Nippon Rinsho 1984;42:2222–7.
4. Nimura Y, Shionoya S. [Diagnosis of bile duct and gallbladder carcinoma by percutaneous transhepatic cholangioscopy]. Gan No Rinsho 1986;32:1246–8.
5. Chen MF, Jan YY, Lee TY. Percutaneous transhepatic cholangioscopy. Br J Surg 1987;74:728–30.
6. Nimura Y, Hayakawa N, Kamiya J, et al. Hepatic segmentectomy with caudate lobe resection for bile duct carcinoma of the hepatic hilus. World J Surg 1990; 14:535–43 [discussion: 544].
7. Nimura Y, Kamiya J, Hayakawa N, et al. Cholangioscopic differentiation of biliary strictures and polyps. Endoscopy 1989;21(Suppl 1):351–6.
8. Nimura Y, Kamiya J, Kondo S, et al. Aggressive preoperative management and extended surgery for hilar cholangiocarcinoma: Nagoya experience. J Hepatobiliary Pancreat Surg 2000;7:155–62.
9. Nimura Y, Shionoya S, Hayakawa N, et al. Value of percutaneous transhepatic cholangioscopy (PTCS). Surg Endosc 1988;2:213–9.
10. Kauffmann GW, Roeren T, Friedl P, et al. Interventional radiological treatment of malignant biliary obstruction. Eur J Surg Oncol 1990;16:397–403.
11. Classen M, Hagenmuller F. Endoprosthesis and local irradiation in the treatment of biliary malignancies. Endoscopy 1987;19(Suppl 1):25–30.
12. Sai JK, Suyama M, Kubokawa Y, et al. Early detection of extrahepatic bile-duct carcinomas in the nonicteric stage by using MRCP followed by EUS. Gastrointest Endosc 2009;70:29–36.
13. Scotiniotis IA, Kochman ML. Intramural cyst of the bile duct demonstrated by cholangioscopy and intraductal US. Gastrointest Endosc 2001;54:260–2.
14. Lu XL, Itoi T, Kubota K. Cholangioscopy by using narrow-band imaging and transpapillary radiotherapy for mucin-producing bile duct tumor. Clin Gastroenterol Hepatol 2009;7:e34–5.
15. Brauer BC, Fukami N, Chen YK. Direct cholangioscopy with narrow-band imaging, chromoendoscopy, and argon plasma coagulation of intraductal papillary mucinous neoplasm of the bile duct (with videos). Gastrointest Endosc 2008;67:574–6.

16. Choi HJ, Moon JH, Ko BM, et al. Overtube-balloon-assisted direct peroral chol-angioscopy by using an ultra-slim upper endoscope (with videos). Gastrointest Endosc 2009;69:935–40.
17. Hochberger J, Tex S, Maiss J, et al. Management of difficult common bile duct stones. Gastrointest Endosc Clin N Am 2003;13:623–34.
18. Hochberger J, Bayer J, May A, et al. Laser lithotripsy of difficult bile duct stones: results in 60 patients using a rhodamine 6G dye laser with optical stone tissue detection system. Gut 1998;43:823–9.
19. Jazrawi SF, Nguyen D, Barnett C, et al. Novel application of intraductal argon plasma coagulation in biliary papillomatosis (with video). Gastrointest Endosc 2009;69:372–4.
20. Suzuki S, Inaba K, Yokoi Y, et al. Photodynamic therapy for malignant biliary obstruction: a case series. Endoscopy 2004;36:83–7.
21. Shim CS, Cheon YK, Cha SW, et al. Prospective study of the effectiveness of percutaneous transhepatic photodynamic therapy for advanced bile duct cancer and the role of intraductal ultrasonography in response assessment. Endoscopy 2005;37:425–33.
22. Sato M, Inoue H, Ogawa S, et al. Limitations of percutaneous transhepatic chol-angioscopy for the diagnosis of the intramural extension of bile duct carcinoma. Endoscopy 1998;30:281–8.

Peroral Pancreatoscopy in the Diagnosis and Management of Intraductal Papillary Mucinous Neoplasia and Indeterminate Pancreatic Duct Pathology

Daniel A. Ringold, MD, Raj J. Shah, MD*

KEYWORDS

- Pancreatoscopy • Intraductal papillary mucinous neoplasia
- Pancreatic duct stricture • Pancreatic adenocarcinoma

Peroral cholangioscopy and peroral pancreatoscopy (POP) are selectively utilized in the evaluation of indeterminate pancreaticobiliary strictures.[1-4] Direct visualization of the pancreatic duct permits the localization of main duct lesions in intraductal papillary mucinous neoplasia (IPMN).[5-7] Although refinement in endoscope technology and technique has permitted wider application of this technology, commercially available devices with a working channel that permits passage of biopsy forceps for tissue acquisition still necessitates an approximately 10-Fr catheter or endoscope system. This requires a dilated pancreatic duct for its use. Whether or not four-way tip deflection enhances maneuverability within the pancreatic duct remains to be established.[8] Prototype electronic pancreatoscopes have improved optical resolution but are limited by fragility and suboptimal working channel diameters.[9,10] The most intriguing application of POP is in the identification and sampling of occult main pancreatic duct (MPD) lesions that may not be visible by noninvasive imaging, transluminal endoscopic ultrasound (EUS), or conventional pancreatography.[11] This review describes how POP may complement existing imaging modalities in the evaluation of patients who have known or suspected IPMN and pancreatic adenocarcinoma.

Division of Gastroenterology and Hepatology, University of Colorado Denver, MS F735, 1635 Aurora Court, Room AIP 2.031, Aurora, CO 80045, USA
* Corresponding author.
E-mail address: raj.shah@ucdenver.edu (R.J. Shah).

Gastrointest Endoscopy Clin N Am 19 (2009) 601–613
doi:10.1016/j.giec.2009.07.002
1052-5157/09/$ – see front matter © 2009 Elsevier Inc. All rights reserved.

giendo.theclinics.com

PERORAL PANCREATOSCOPY EQUIPMENT AND TECHNIQUE

In-depth evaluations of the different cholangiopancreatoscopes are in articles by Kelsey and Chen elsewhere in this issue and in a recent technical review by the American Society of Gastrointestinal Endoscopy's Technology Committee.[11] One of the notable emerging advances with this technology includes video cholangiopancreatoscopes that use charge-coupled devices in their tips to generate high-definition digital images of the pancreatic duct, representing a significant enhancement in optics over the conventional fiberoptic devices.[12] Narrow band imaging (NBI) enhancement technology (Olympus Medical Systems, Tokyo, Japan), provided by a videocholangioscope that has a 3.4-mm outer diameter, improves vascular pattern detection of tumor vessels (dilated, tortuous blood vessels) and possibly mucosal pathology.[13,14] The semidisposable SpyGlass Direct Visualization System (Boston Scientific, Natick, MA) incorporates four-way tip deflection that potentially improves maneuverability within the duct. Two dedicated ports for irrigation and aspiration may enhance the clearance of thick mucin, proteinaceous debris, and stone fragments that often obscure intraductal inspection.[8,15]

Depending on anatomy, POP is feasible through the major or minor papilla. POP access through the minor papilla, however, is technically challenging because of a very short or long duodenoscope position that is required for device introduction. This may limit maneuverability and endosocope stability.

The technique of performing POP is similar to that of cholangioscopy with the caveat that for commercially available devices, the depth of endoscope insertion within the pancreatic duct may be limited because of downstream tortuous segments (eg, genu and pancreatic head) and/or narrower ducts (5 mm or less). In the absence of a patulous orifice seen with MPD-IPMN, pancreatic sphincterotomy is required.[16] Further, the authors tend to reduce the force and volume of intraductal irrigation to help minimize the risk of postprocedural pancreatitis.

POP can provide directed tissue sampling through the 1.2- to 2.6-mm accessory channels of currently available cholangioscopes. If passage of the biopsy forceps is not possible because of a tortuous endoscope position, POP-assisted biopsies can be performed. With this technique, a fluoroscopic spot film of the pancreatoscope at the point of interest guides tissue sampling through the accessory channel of the duodenoscope under fluoroscopy guidance.[2] A more detailed review of tissue sampling methods and efficacy can be found in the article by Pleskow elsewhere in this issue.

INTRADUCTAL PAPILLARY MUCINOUS NEOPLASIA

Since Ohashi and colleagues first described them in 1982, IPMN are increasingly recognized as mucin-producing tumors of variable malignant potential that involve the pancreatic duct mucosa.[17] Three distinct forms have been described: MPD-IPMN, side-branch pancreatic duct (SB-IPMN), and involveing MPD and SB (mixed IPMN). The risk of high-grade dysplasia or malignancy in patients who have MPD lesions is approximately 60% compared with approximately 20% in patients with SB lesions.[17–19] Thus, determining the presence of MPD involvement in patients with a dilated duct and suspected IPMN is clinically important.[19–23] IPMNs seem multifocal in approximately 20% of cases, often contributing to the difficulty in obtaining clear surgical margins.[24] IPMNs often are discovered incidentally on imaging studies, such as CT or magnetic resonance cholangiopancreatography (MRCP). With MPD-IPMN, imaging studies typically demonstrate a dilated pancreatic duct and, in the case of SB-IPMN, may suggest cystic pancreatic lesions that communicate with a side branch.[25] Although CT and MRCP studies are helpful in the detection of cystic pancreatic lesions, distinguishing ductal dilation of IPMN from chronic pancreatitis or SB-IPMN from pseudocysts or determining whether or not a pancreatic cyst communicates with the pancreatic duct is limited.[26] Histologically, IPMNs occur in a spectrum from adenoma to adenocarcinoma and are believed to progress to advanced histology in a manner analogous to colon polyps. Histology or cytology from an IPMN demonstrating high-grade dysplasia or invasive carcinoma necessitates surgical resection or chemotherapy.[27]

As with other neoplastic processes, accurate tissue sampling and definition of disease extent are paramount to appropriate management of IPMN. Endoscopic retrograde cholangiopancreatography (ERCP) and EUS with fine-needle aspiration (FNA) are the most commonly used modalities to establish the diagnosis of IPMN.[28,29] During ERCP for suspected MPD-IPMN, a pathognomonic fish-mouth papilla exuding mucin may be seen in approximately 40% of cases, and on pancreatography, the MPD often is cystically dilated and filled with mucin (see **Fig. 1**).[19,30] Pancreatography alone, however, may be less sensitive than MRCP in identifying intraductal nodules or masses that would assist in localizing tissue sampling attempts or determining resection margins.[17,31] EUS with FNA permits the identification and sampling of mural nodules and provides information on endosonographic features, cytology, and cyst fluid tumor markers to assist in establishing a diagnosis.[32,33] Some studies suggest, however, that cytology from pancreatic cysts has marginal utility in assessing the presence and degree of dysplasia present within a lesion, with sensitivities as low as 50% in distinguishing malignant from nonmalignant lesions.[32–35]

As a result of the limited sensitivity of the available diagnostic modalities, clinical features, such as weight loss, jaundice, and abdominal pain, along with imaging characteristics (size, mural nodules, and masses) often are relied on to estimate the risk of malignancy and to determine the plan for surgical resection versus surveillance. In surgically fit patients, resection is indicated if symptoms are present, there is MPD involvement (including the mixed subtype), or if malignant potential remains indeterminate.[27]

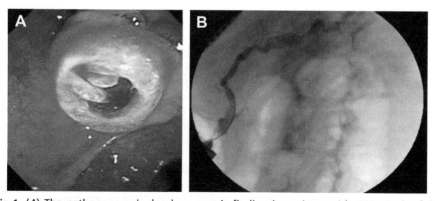

Fig. 1. (A) The pathognomonic duodeonoscopic finding in patients with IPMN is the fish-mouth papilla exuding mucin. (B) The pancreatographic findings of IPMN are a dilated pancreatic duct with filling defects and underfilling of the duct due to excessive amounts of mucin.

Earlier diagnostic strategies for IPMN resulted in inaccurate preoperative disease localization. In a series of 47 patients who had IPMN undergoing surgical resection, CT, EUS, and ERCP were only 62% accurate in predicting the lateral spread of MPD-IPMN and only 80% accurate in detecting malignancy resulting in positive surgical margins for 41% of patients.[36] An approximately 50% postoperative recurrence rate may have been partly the result of inaccurate preoperative staging and IPMN's frequent multifocal nature.[24,37,38] POP may potentially complement these other modalities by detecting unsuspected high-risk features, such as mass lesions and tumors vessels, or determining the extent of disease in MPD-IPMN and the presence of main duct disease in suspected mixed IPMN.

PERORAL PANCREATOSCOPY FINDINGS IN PATIENTS WITH INTRADUCTAL PAPILLARY MUCINOUS NEOPLASIA

Early descriptions of intraductal findings by POP in patients who had IPMN included mucin, papillary projections in the main duct or from a side branch, and subtle mucosal nodular changes.[5–7,39–41] The histologic continuum of IPMN that exists has not been elucidated until recently, however. In an elegant description of the pancreatoscopic spectrum of IPMN in patients undergoing surgical resection, Hara and colleagues reviewed their experience with 60 patients, some of whom underwent concomitant intraductal ultrasound (IDUS).[42] There were 23 patients who had MPD lesions and 37 who had SB lesions who had previously undergone CT and EUS with lesions noted in the pancreatic head (N = 44), body (N = 10), and tail (N = 6). POP findings included the presence and extent of duct wall irregularity, tumor vessels, and the morphology of protruding lesions. Using IDUS, the height of the projections or nodules was measured and the lesions were divided into five progressive subtypes based on the height and appearance of the projections: (1) granular, (2) fish-egg, (3) fish-egg with prominent vasculature, (4) villous, and (5) vegetative types (see **Fig. 2**). The investigators demonstrated that projections at least 4 mm in height, as determined by IDUS, were more likely (88%) to be carcinoma in situ or invasive carcinoma than smaller projections. POP inspection alone was 68% sensitive, 87% specific, and 75% accurate in the detection of malignancy. POP was more accurate for MPD lesions whereas IDUS proved superior for SB lesions. The combination of POP and IDUS was 88% accurate in differentiating benign from malignant lesions and was higher than CT, EUS, POP, and IDUS alone. IPMN subtypes 3, 4, and 5 contained carcinoma in situ or adenocarcinoma in approximately 90% of cases compared to 0% of subtypes 1 and 2. Within this framework of the progressive POP appearance of IPMN, subtype 3 lesions containing prominent vasculature are likely the earliest marker of advanced histology. The presence of subtypes 3, 4, and 5 should raise concern for malignancy and prompt referral for resection. Remarkably, only one patient (1.7%) had a positive surgical margin and, although not subsequently reproduced, does suggest the value of preoperative POP and IDUS in the management of IPMN. Intraoperative pancreatoscopy also seems to assist in determining the extent of resection necessary to attain negative surgical margins. In a series of 24 patients who underwent intraoperative pancreatoscopy, there were no positive margins or tumor recurrences at a mean follow-up of 4 years.[43] The investigators noted that one of the advantages of this method was the ability to manually manipulate the pancreas to facilitate pancreatoscope passage and mucosal inspection.

An additional series of patients undergoing POP included 60 patients who had surgically confirmed IPMN of whom 57 (95%) underwent technically successful POP. The reasons for the three cases of POP failures and the distribution of the lesions were not

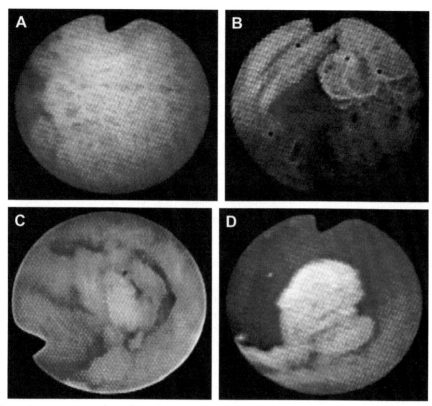

Fig. 2. Pancreatoscopy has allowed endoscopists to visualize the entire spectrum of intraductal papillary mucinous neoplasms. Four of the forms are demonstrated: (*A*) granular, (*B*) fish-egg, (*C*) villous projection, and (*D*) vegetative nodule.

specified. POP findings included papillary projections (58%), mucin only (23%), granular mucosa (16%), and coarse mucosa (4%). Papillary projections were more prevalent in cases that demonstrated more aggressive histology (23% of adenoma, 58% of borderline, 70% of noninvasive IPMN, and 89% of invasive IPMN).[4] No comment was made, however, regarding the height of papillary projections or the presence of prominent vasculature and their relationship to malignant transformation. In a smaller series of 12 patients who had IPMN (11 MPD, 1 SB), the investigators observed oval-shaped, fish-egg lesions in 10 patients and nodular or villous changes in two patients. The patients who had invasive IPMN consisted of the oval-shaped tumors with erythema or villous tumors and dilated blood (tumor) vessels. In the one case of SB-IPMN, POP observed papillary projections spreading from the orifice of the affected side branch.[10]

At the authors' center, POP has been found useful in localizing MPD-IPMN, excluding lesions in the head for anticipated extended pancreatic tail resection, and evaluating for mixed IPMN in patients with established SB-IPMN. Preliminarily, 11 patients withIPMN (7 MPD IPMN and 4 SB-IPMN) have been evaluated.[44] The POP findings in seven patients who had MPD IPMN included a vegetative mass and villous projections (N = 1), villous projections and mucin (N = 5), and mucin alone (N = 1). The POP findings in the four patients with SB-IPMN included a dilated MPD in two, mucin in one, and a fibrotic-appearing duct in one patient. Six patients underwent POP-directed and -assisted biopsies and histology confirmed malignant (N = 1) and nonmalignant (N = 5) IPMN.

For IPMN, POP-assisted pancreatic juice aspiration for cytology also has been described. Although there are limited data on this technique, the method requires saline lavage of the MPD with direct aspiration of pancreatic juice through the pancreatoscope channel. One study assessed 103 consecutive patients who underwent surgical resection for IPMN.[45] All patients had pancreatic juice cytology and the investigators compared catheter-based secretin-enhanced collection with POP-based pancreatic juice aspiration and found that the POP-based method had higher sensitivity that did not reach statistical significance (62% versus 38%; P = 0.055) for the detection of IPMN. In the patient population, 76 of 103 (74%) patients had SB-IPMN but whether or not these were mixed-type IPMN was not specified. Overall, pancreatic juice cytology was able to detect 50% of confirmed malignant IPMN.[45] The technique seems a useful adjunct to POP but may be of limited value in determining the extent of surgical resection.

INDETERMINATE PANCREATIC DUCT STRICTURES AND DUCTAL ADENOCARINOMA

At the time of diagnosis, most pancreatic adenocarcinomas are unresectable. Of those patients who undergo apparent curative resection, median and 5-year survival is only 18 to 20 months and 10% to 25%, respectively. The best outcome is seen in patients who have small, well-differentiated tumors without retroperitoneal invasion or lymph node metastases; thus, the early diagnosis of pancreatic cancers may improve survival.[46] Patients in pancreatic cancer families and those with hereditary chronic pancreatitis are at the highest risk for the development of pancreatic adenocarcinoma.[47,48] Epidemiologic studies suggest an approximately 15-fold increase in risk in patients with nonfamilial chronic pancreatitis.[49] Although the majority of pancreatic duct strictures in patients chronic pancreatitis are benign, early pancreatic cancers or pancreatic intraepethelial neoplasia can present as isolated MPD strictures in up to 12% of cases.[50] EUS has a high diagnostic yield in identifying and sampling masses in the pancreas that may not be detected by noninvasive imaging.[51,52] The yield of EUS-FNA in patients with chronic pancreatitis and isolated ductal strictures, however, seems lower.[53] Conventional ERCP tissue sampling in the pancreatic duct is limited by variable sensitivity of brush cytology and difficulty in advancing biopsy forceps to an area of interest.[54-56]

Direct intraductal inspection may enhance the diagnosis of malignancy. For biliary strictures, cholangioscopy improves the diagnostic accuracy of tissue sampling; however, randomized studies comparing cholangioscopy to conventional ERCP techniques are lacking.[2] Cholangioscopy can detect the presence of dilated, tortuous tumor vessels and, when combined with visually directed biopsies, has demonstrated a sensitivity of 96% in detecting malignancy.[57] Anatomic differences between the biliary and pancreatic ductal systems may yield different results in evaluating indeterminate pancreatic duct pathology.

PERORAL PANCREATOSCOPY FINDINGS IN INDETERMINATE PANCREATIC DUCT STRICTURES

Studies of POP for strictures are primarily uncontrolled, small case series. In one of the earliest series on POP, Tajiri and colleagues reported the use of ultrathin pancreatoscopes (0.8 mm) primarily without sphincterotomy to evaluate normal subjects (n = 25) and patients with pancreatic disease (n = 27).[58] Among these 52 subjects, POP was able to reach the target lesion or pancreatic tail in 42 (81%) cases. Among the 10 failed cases, the pancreatoscope could not traverse the papilla in five or be advanced to the tail because of angulations of the duct in five. Pancreatic duct strictures were identified in 22 (52%) and the remaining 20 examinations were normal. POP findings in the seven malignant strictures were friability and erythema (100%), nodularity (71%), and erosive changes (57%). For the 15 benign strictures, findings included a scarred appearance and ductal erythema. Another case series of 56 subjects included 13 IPMN, 8 pancreatic adenocarcinomas, 32 benign chronic pancreatitis patients, and 3 normal examinations. In the eight patients who had adenocarcinoma, POP adequately visualized strictures in five of them. Characteristics included friable, erythematous mucosa (N = 4) and extrinsic compression of normal mucosa (N = 1). Patients with benign strictures had scarred-appearing or edematous mucosa.[10]

Yamao and colleagues reported the largest series of POP for indeterminate pancreatic duct strictures, evaluating a total of 55 patients who underwent intraductal inspection without apparent directed tissue sampling.[4] Indications for POP included suspected chronic pancreatitis and abnormal ductal findings on imaging studies. EUS was performed in an unspecified number of subjects prior to POP. Malignancy was determined by surgical pathology whereas benign strictures were followed for a minimum of 2 years. Thirty-five strictures were histologically confirmed as malignant and 20 as benign. Only 22 (63%) of the malignant and 16 (80%) of the benign strictures, however, could be observed directly with POP. Among the malignant strictures, the POP findings were coarse mucosa (59%), friability (50%), erythema alone (36%), protrusion (27%), tumor vessels (23%), and papillary projections (14%). In contrast, benign strictures were noted to have a smooth stenosis (62%), erythema (25%), and coarse mucosa (13%). Of all of the POP findings, coarse mucosa and friability had the highest sensitivities for malignancy of 59% and 50%, respectively, whereas protrusion, friability, tumor vessels, and papillary projections each had a specificity of 100% for malignancy. The presence of erythema alone was nonspecific.

In the authors' experience with POP for MPD strictures, a total of 24 patients (20 benign and 4 adenocarcinoma) were evaluated in the past 8 years.[44] These procedures were performed mainly to evaluate ductal dilation. In two of the four patients who had adenocarcinoma, nodularity or protrusions were seen. In the other two patients, smooth strictures with normal-appearing mucosa could not be traversed with the pancreatoscope, and diagnosis subsequently was made by EUS and surgical exploration, respectively. Among the 20 benign strictures, 11 appeared scarred and 9 had erythema. None of the benign-appearing strictures had more concerning findings, such as nodularity or protrusion (see **Fig. 3**). The patients with presumed benign strictures were followed for a mean of 31 months without a subsequent cancer diagnosis.

Ideally, POP would enable physicians to diagnose pancreatic cancer at its earliest possible stage. Few data exist, however, on the diagnosis of these early tumors. In a case series, Uehara and colleagues reported the successful diagnosis of pancreatic carcinoma in situ by POP in 11 patients.[59] All of the patients had previously undergone extensive diagnostic work-ups, consisting of CT, EUS, and ERCP without a definitive diagnosis. On POP, the investigators observed papillary, irregular, and nodular mucosa in the MPD. In addition to POP, pancreatic juice was collected by the catheter- and pancreatoscopy-based methods. The catheter-based method was diagnostic in 60% of cases compared to 100% with the pancreatoscopy-based method. Although encouraging, its small sample size and lack of control group limits its wider application.

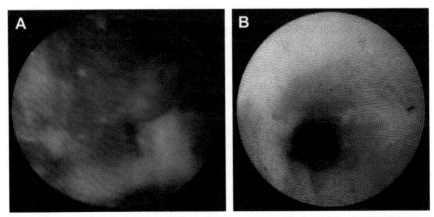

Fig. 3. (A) This malignant stricture demonstrates an infiltrative appearance. (B) This benign stricture has a smooth, scarred appearance.

LIMITATIONS AND SAFETY OF PERORAL PANCREATOSCOPY IN PATIENTS WITH INTRADUCTAL PAPILLARY MUCINOUS NEOPLASIA AND DUCTAL STRICTURES

Anatomic factors that may limit the successful completion of pancreatoscopy include a narrow caliber duct, tight strictures, downstream tortuosity, and obstructing stones. Careful pre-inspection stricture dilation may improve access but resultant mucosal bleeding compromises visualization. Smaller-caliber pancreatoscopes may overcome these barriers; however, they only permit inspection without directed tissue sampling. Using stiffer guide wires may enhance the ability to provide back-tension for negotiating circuitous segments. A fixed pancreatoscope tip position from reduced maneuverability across tortuous segments may limit circumferential inspection. Applying torque on the duodenoscope, however, may help improve visualization. Whether or not the semidisposable cholangioscope with four-way tip deflection will provide improved maneuverability within the pancreatic duct remains to be established.

Aside from maneuverability, a limitation of POP in patients with IPMN is the obscured view from thick intraductal mucin despite irrigation and suction. Inspection may be enhanced in this scenario if balloon extraction of mucin is performed prior to pancreatoscope insertion. Another option is to lavage and aspirate the MPD with sterile saline in an attempt to break up and remove the mucin. In cases when adequate ductal clearance of mucin cannot be achieved by these methods, the authors' group has used a dilute solution of the mucolytic agent, N-acetylcysteine, to successfully improve visualization.[60] Although POP has its limitations, careful patient selection and operator experience are important factors in enhancing efficacy.

With respect to complications from POP, few comprehensive data exist. In the largest series, the reported frequency of POP-related pancreatitis ranged from 1% to 12%.[4,8,42] In the absence of a patulous pancreatic orifice in the setting of IPMN, pancreatic sphincterotomy often is required. If downstream ductal strictures are identified, careful pre-POP balloon dilatation is necessary to reach the target depth of insertion. Ultrathin pancreatoscopes also may be used but are not commercially available and lack an accessory channel.

If a prolonged procedure is anticipated, the authors recommend performing POP with general anesthesia. Due to intraductal sterile saline lavage to improve inspection, risk of pulmonary aspiration secondary to reflux of fluid into the stomach exists but may be reduced by thorough suctioning prior to duodenoscope withdrawal.[11] Although no cases of bacteremia or pancreatic sepsis have been reported with POP, the authors' preference is to administer prophylactic antibiotics.

FUTURE TRENDS IN PERORAL PANCREATOSCOPY

Although advances in miniature endoscope technology have permitted improved image resolution, maneuverability, and durability, an ideal device that has incorporated each of these enhanced features is lacking. Refinements in endoscope caliber, image quality, and tip deflection are still required. Further miniaturization of the pancreatoscope without sacrificing image quality and enhancing digital imaging, such as the addition of NBI, are encouraging areas of investigation. In early studies, NBI has provided high-contrast imaging of the pancreatic duct and the detection of IPMN, inflammatory pancreatic lesions, and more subtle pancreatic duct lesions.[61] Furthermore, it provides excellent visualization of vascular patterns and tumor vessels that are harbingers of malignancy.[61,62] One of the limitations with NBI is that blood from trauma or tissue sampling is opaque and obscures visualization when the NBI setting is selected. Furthermore, tip deflection has similar limitations to conventional fiberoptic cholangioscopes. The recently developed ultrathin catheterscope uses a single optical fiber for laser light illumination and few fibers for light collection. The single illumination fiber vibrates and replaces the need for multiple illumination fibers while providing high-quality color video. These features allow the shaft of the endoscope to be only 1.2 mm in diameter and remain highly flexible. Preliminary data in a swine model demonstrated encouraging image resolution but human data are awaited.[63] Maintaining reasonable costs and device durability for all of these advances in technology needs to be considered and may continue to limit widespread availability.

SUMMARY

POP is an exciting modality for the evaluation of pancreatic diseases. It has proven efficacy in the evaluation of suspected IPMN and allows for a determination of the extent of pancreatic duct involvement. POP seems to be a useful adjunct in the evaluation of indeterminate pancreatic duct strictures when other imaging studies are inconclusive. POP has the distinct advantage of allowing tissue acquisition under direct vision, which increases its sensitivity. Further refinement in endoscope caliber, tip deflection, and optics are required for more routine application in pancreatic diseases.

REFERENCES

1. Siddique I, Galati J, Ankoma-Sey V, et al. The role of choledochoscopy in the diagnosis and management of biliary tract diseases. Gastrointest Endosc 1999; 50(1):67–73.
2. Shah RJ, Langer DA, Antillon MR, et al. Cholangioscopy and cholangioscopic forceps biopsy in patients with indeterminate pancreaticobiliary pathology. Clin Gastroenterol Hepatol 2006;4(2):219–25.
3. Tischendorf JJ, Kruger M, Trautwein C, et al. Cholangioscopic characterization of dominant bile duct stenoses in patients with primary sclerosing cholangitis. Endoscopy 2006;38(7):665–9.
4. Yamao K, Ohashi K, Nakamura T, et al. Efficacy of peroral pancreatoscopy in the diagnosis of pancreatic diseases. Gastrointest Endosc 2003;57(2):205–9.

5. Schoonbroodt D, Zipf A, Herrmann G, et al. Pancreatoscopy and diagnosis of mucinous neoplasms of the pancreas. Gastrointest Endosc 1996;44(4):479–82.

6. Koshitani T, Kodama T, Sato H, et al. Clinical application of the peroral electronic pancreatoscope for the investigation of intraductal mucin-hypersecreting neoplasm. Gastrointest Endosc 2000;52(1):95–9.

7. Seo DW, Kim MH, Lee SK, et al. The value of pancreatoscopy in patients with mucinous ductal ectasia. Endoscopy 1997;29(4):315–8.

8. Chen YK, Tarnasky PR, Raijman I, et al. Peroral pancreatoscopy (PP) for pancreatic stone therapy and investigation of susptected pancreatic lesions—first human experience using the Spyglass Direct Visualization System (SDVS) [abstract]. Gastrointest Endosc 2008;67(5):108.

9. Kodama T, Sato H, Horii Y, et al. Pancreatoscopy for the next generation: development of the peroral electronic pancreatoscope system. Gastrointest Endosc 1999;49(3 Pt 1):366–71.

10. Kodama T, Koshitani T, Sato H, et al. Electronic pancreatoscopy for the diagnosis of pancreatic diseases. Am J Gastroenterol 2002;97(3):617–22.

11. Shah RJ, Adler DG, Conway JD, et al. Cholangiopancreatoscopy: ASGE Technology Committee Status Evaluation Report. Gastrointest Endosc 2008;68(3): 411–21.

12. Kodama T, Tatsumi Y, Sato H, et al. Initial experience with a new peroral electronic pancreatoscope with an accessory channel. Gastrointest Endosc 2004;59(7): 895–900.

13. Itoi T, Sofuni A, Itokawa F, et al. Peroral cholangioscopic diagnosis of biliary-tract diseases by using narrow-band imaging (with videos). Gastrointest Endosc 2007; 66(4):730–6.

14. Shah RJ, Chen YK. Video cholangiopancreatoscopy with narrow band imaging: spectrum of mucosal and vascular patterns in patients with pancreaticobiliary pathology [abstract]. Gastrointest Endosc 2009;68(5):AB117.

15. Chen YK, Pleskow DK. SpyGlass single-operator peroral cholangiopancreatoscopy system for the diagnosis and therapy of bile-duct disorders: a clinical feasibility study (with video). Gastrointest Endosc 2007;65(6):832–41.

16. Shah RJ, Chen YK. Techniques of peroral and percutaneous choledochoscopy for evaluation and treatment of biliary stones and strictures. Tech Gastrointest Endosc 2007;9(3):161–8.

17. Ohashi K, Murakami Y, Maruyama M. Four cases of a mucous secreting pancreatic cancer. Prog Dig Endosc 1982;20:348–51.

18. Levy P, Jouannaud V, O'Toole D, et al. Natural history of intraductal papillary mucinous tumors of the pancreas: actuarial risk of malignancy. Clin Gastroenterol Hepatol 2006;4(4):460–8.

19. Suzuki Y, Atomi Y, Sugiyama M, et al. Cystic neoplasm of the pancreas: a Japanese multiinstitutional study of intraductal papillary mucinous tumor and mucinous cystic tumor. Pancreas 2004;28(3):241–6.

20. Kobari M, Egawa S, Shibuya K, et al. Intraductal papillary mucinous tumors of the pancreas comprise 2 clinical subtypes: differences in clinical characteristics and surgical management. Arch Surg 1999;134(10):1131–6.

21. Terris B, Ponsot P, Paye F, et al. Intraductal papillary mucinous tumors of the pancreas confined to secondary ducts show less aggressive pathologic features as compared with those involving the main pancreatic duct. Am J Surg Pathol 2000;24(10):1372–7.

22. Doi R, Fujimoto K, Wada M, et al. Surgical management of intraductal papillary mucinous tumor of the pancreas. Surgery 2002;132(1):80–5.

23. Kitagawa Y, Unger TA, Taylor S, et al. Mucus is a predictor of better prognosis and survival in patients with intraductal papillary mucinous tumor of the pancreas. J Gastrointest Surg 2003;7(1):12–8.
24. Rodriguez JR, Salvia R, Crippa S, et al. Branch-duct intraductal papillary mucinous neoplasms: observations in 145 patients who underwent resection. Gastroenterology 2007;133(1):72–9.
25. Kim YH, Saini S, Sahani D, et al. Imaging diagnosis of cystic pancreatic lesions: pseudocyst versus nonpseudocyst. Radiographics 2005;25(3):671–85.
26. Procacci C, Megibow AJ, Carbognin G, et al. Intraductal papillary mucinous tumor of the pancreas: a pictorial essay. Radiographics 1999;19(6):1447–63.
27. Khalid A, Brugge W. ACG practice guidelines for the diagnosis and management of neoplastic pancreatic cysts. Am J Gastroenterol 2007;102(10):2339–49.
28. Baba T, Yamaguchi T, Ishihara T, et al. Distinguishing benign from malignant intraductal papillary mucinous tumors of the pancreas by imaging techniques. Pancreas 2004;29(3):212–7.
29. Yamao K, Ohashi K, Nakamura T, et al. Evaluation of various imaging methods in the differential diagnosis of intraductal papillary-mucinous tumor (IPMT) of the pancreas. Hepatogastroenterology 2001;48(40):962–6.
30. Yamaguchi K, Tanaka M. Mucin-hypersecreting tumor of the pancreas with mucin extrusion through an enlarged papilla. Am J Gastroenterol 1991;86(7):835–9.
31. Yamaguchi K, Ogawa Y, Chijiiwa K, et al. Mucin-hypersecreting tumors of the pancreas: assessing the grade of malignancy preoperatively. Am J Surg 1996; 171(4):427–31.
32. Frossard JL, Amouyal P, Amouyal G, et al. Performance of endosonography-guided fine needle aspiration and biopsy in the diagnosis of pancreatic cystic lesions. Am J Gastroenterol 2003;98(7):1516–24.
33. Bhutani MS. Role of endoscopic ultrasonography in the diagnosis and treatment of cystic tumors of the pancreas. JOP 2004;5(4):266–72.
34. Pais SA, Attasaranya S, Leblanc JK, et al. Role of endoscopic ultrasound in the diagnosis of intraductal papillary mucinous neoplasms: correlation with surgical histopathology. Clin Gastroenterol Hepatol 2007;5(4):489–95.
35. Emerson RE, Randolph ML, Cramer HM. Endoscopic ultrasound-guided fine-needle aspiration cytology diagnosis of intraductal papillary mucinous neoplasm of the pancreas is highly predictive of pancreatic neoplasia. Diagn Cytopathol 2006;34(7):457–62.
36. Cellier C, Cuillerier E, Palazzo L, et al. Intraductal papillary and mucinous tumors of the pancreas: accuracy of preoperative computed tomography, endoscopic retrograde pancreatography and endoscopic ultrasonography, and long-term outcome in a large surgical series. Gastrointest Endosc 1998; 47(1):42–9.
37. Sho M, Nakajima Y, Kanehiro H, et al. Pattern of recurrence after resection for intraductal papillary mucinous tumors of the pancreas. World J Surg 1998;22(8): 874–8.
38. Azar C, Van de Stadt J, Rickaert F, et al. Intraductal papillary mucinous tumours of the pancreas. Clinical and therapeutic issues in 32 patients. Gut 1996;39(3): 457–64.
39. Mukai H, Yasuda K, Nakajima M. Differential diagnosis of mucin-producing tumors of the pancreas by intraductal ultrasonography and peroral pancreatoscopy. Endoscopy 1998;30(Suppl 1):A99–102.
40. Fujita N, Lee SI, Kobayashi G, et al. Pancreatoscopy for mucus producing pancreatic tumor. Dig Endosc 1990;2:110–5.

41. Yamao K, Nakazawa S, Naito Y, et al. The efficacy of peroral transpapillary pancreatoscopy (POPS) for the diagnosis of mucus-producing pancreatic tumors. Gastrointest Endosc 1988;30:563–9.
42. Hara T, Yamaguchi T, Ishihara T, et al. Diagnosis and patient management of intraductal papillary-mucinous tumor of the pancreas by using peroral pancreatoscopy and intraductal ultrasonography. Gastroenterology 2002;122(1): 34–43.
43. Kaneko T, Nakao A, Nomoto S, et al. Intraoperative pancreatoscopy with the ultrathin pancreatoscope for mucin-producing tumors of the pancreas. Arch Surg 1998;133(3):263–7.
44. Ringold DA, Shah RJ, Yen RD, et al. The role of peroral pancreatoscopy in the evaluation of main pancreatic duct neoplasia. Gastrointest Endosc 2009;68(5). [abstract].
45. Yamaguchi T, Shirai Y, Ishihara T, et al. Pancreatic juice cytology in the diagnosis of intraductal papillary mucinous neoplasm of the pancreas: significance of sampling by peroral pancreatoscopy. Cancer 2005;104(12):2830–6.
46. Sener SF, Fremgen A, Menck HR, et al. Pancreatic cancer: a report of treatment and survival trends for 100,313 patients diagnosed from 1985–1995, using the National Cancer Database. J Am Coll Surg 1999;189(1):1–7.
47. Lowenfels AB, Maisonneuve P, Whitcomb DC. Risk factors for cancer in hereditary pancreatitis. International Hereditary Pancreatitis Study Group. Med Clin North Am 2000;84(3):565–73.
48. Whitcomb DC, Applebaum S, Martin SP. Hereditary pancreatitis and pancreatic carcinoma. Ann N Y Acad Sci 1999;880:201–9.
49. Lowenfels AB, Maisonneuve P, Cavallini G, et al. Pancreatitis and the risk of pancreatic cancer. International Pancreatitis Study Group. N Engl J Med 1993; 328(20):1433–7.
50. Kalady MF, Peterson B, Baillie J, et al. Pancreatic duct strictures: identifying risk of malignancy. Ann Surg Oncol 2004;11(6):581–8.
51. Agarwal B, Abu-Hamda E, Molke KL, et al. Endoscopic ultrasound-guided fine needle aspiration and multidetector spiral CT in the diagnosis of pancreatic cancer. Am J Gastroenterol 2004;99(5):844–50.
52. Klapman JB, Chang KJ, Lee JG, et al. Negative predictive value of endoscopic ultrasound in a large series of patients with a clinical suspicion of pancreatic cancer. Am J Gastroenterol 2005;100(12):2658–61.
53. Krishna NB, Mehra M, Reddy AV, et al. EUS/EUS-FNA for suspected pancreatic cancer: influence of chronic pancreatitis and clinical presentation with or without obstructive jaundice on performance characteristics. Gastrointest Endosc 2009; 70(1):70.
54. Athanassiadou P, Grapsa D. Value of endoscopic retrograde cholangiopancreatography-guided brushings in preoperative assessment of pancreaticobiliary strictures: what's new? Acta Cytol 2008;52(1):24–34.
55. Elek G, Gyokeres T, Schafer E, et al. Early diagnosis of pancreatobiliary duct malignancies by brush cytology and biopsy. Pathol Oncol Res 2005;11(3):145–55.
56. McGuire DE, Venu RP, Brown RD, et al. Brush cytology for pancreatic carcinoma: an analysis of factors influencing results. Gastrointest Endosc 1996;44(3):300–4.
57. Kim HJ, Kim MH, Lee SK, et al. Tumor vessel: a valuable cholangioscopic clue of malignant biliary stricture. Gastrointest Endosc 2000;52(5):635–8.
58. Tajiri H, Kobayashi M, Niwa H, et al. Clinical application of an ultra-thin pancreatoscope using a sequential video converter. Gastrointest Endosc 1993;39(3): 371–4.

59. Uehara H, Nakaizumi A, Tatsuta M, et al. Diagnosis of carcinoma in situ of the pancreas by peroral pancreatoscopy and pancreatoscopic cytology. Cancer 1997;79(3):454–61.
60. Brauer BC, Fukami N, Chen YK. Direct cholangioscopy with narrow-band imaging, chromoendoscopy, and argon plasma coagulation of intraductal papillary mucinous neoplasm of the bile duct (with videos). Gastrointest Endosc 2008; 67(3):574–6.
61. Itoi T, Sofuni A, Itokawa F, et al. Initial experience of peroral pancreatoscopy combined with narrow-band imaging in the diagnosis of intraductal papillary mucinous neoplasms of the pancreas (with videos). Gastrointest Endosc 2007; 66(4):793–7.
62. Tanaka K, Yasuda K, Uno K, et al. Evaluation of narrow band imaging for peroral cholangiopancreatoscopy. Digestive Endoscopy 2007;19(Suppl 1):S129–33.
63. Seibel E, Melville C, Johnston R, et al. Bile duct imaging with ultrathin laser scanning catheterscope in a swine model. Gastrointest Endosc 2008;67(5):AB133–4.

Clinical Application of Intraductal Ultrasound During Endoscopic Retrograde Cholangiopancreatography

Rabi Kundu, MD[a], Douglas Pleskow, MD[b],*

KEYWORDS

- Intraductal ultrasound • ERCP • Biliary diseases
- Pancreatic diseases

Biliary and pancreatic diseases may be difficult to diagnose. Transabdominal ultrasound (US), computed tomography (CT), Magnetic resonance cholangiopancreatography (MRCP), endoscopic ultrasound (EUS), and endoscopic retrograde cholangiopancreatography (ERCP) are the traditional imaging modalities commonly used in the evaluation of biliary and pancreatic disorders. These imaging modalities may be less reliable in the evaluation of some difficult biliopancreatic disorders. Intraductal ultrasound (IDUS) used during ERCP can facilitate in the evaluation of these disorders.

US probes can be introduced through the working channel of a duodenoscope and passed selectively into both the biliary and pancreatic ducts. US frequencies of 20 or 30 MHz enable a penetration of up to 2 cm and a resolution of 0.07 to 0.18 mm. EUS probes are available in various diameters (2–2.9 mm), frequencies (12–30 MHz), and lengths (170–220 cm). Higher US frequency yields higher resolution at the expense of reduced depth of penetration. The average depths of penetration are 29 mm for the 12-MHz probe and 18 mm for the 20-MHz probe.[1] One probe is designed for the passage over a guide wire to facilitate use in pancreas and bile ducts. The acoustic coupling in the biliary and pancreatic duct is optimized by the tubular anatomy of both ducts, which are fluid-filled and normally are slightly larger in diameter than the probe itself. The experience of IDUS was first reported by Martin and colleagues and Silverstein and colleagues in 1989.[2,3] The smaller diameter, flexibility, and the image quality

---

[a] Division of Gastroenterology, UCSF Fresno, 2823 Fresno Street, 1st Floor Endoscopy Suite, Fresno, CA 93721, USA
[b] Division of Gastroenterology, Beth Israel Deaconess Medical Center, Harvard Medical School, 110 Frances Street, 8E, Boston, MA 02215, USA
* Corresponding author.
E-mail address: dpleskow@bidmc.harvard.edu (D. Pleskow).

Gastrointest Endoscopy Clin N Am 19 (2009) 615–628
doi:10.1016/j.giec.2009.06.004
1052-5157/09/$ – see front matter © 2009 Elsevier Inc. All rights reserved.

offered by these devices makes them ideal for evaluating a variety of difficult biliary and pancreatic diseases, especially in undefined strictures, luminal filling defects, and ampullary neoplasms (**Table 1**).

TECHNICAL CONSIDERATIONS

Three intraductal ultrasound systems has been developed: (1) electronic cylindrical phased array, (2) combined (radial and linear scanning), and (3) mechanical radial sector scan. The electronic cylindrical phased array uses 1.2-mm catheters with no rotating parts, and is extremely flexible. There are 64 transducer elements, which produce a 360° image. This system has a poor lateral resolution (about one-fifth) as compared with the mechanical systems. The commonly used transducer is a mechanical probe, which has a single transducer, a cable to rotate the transducer, a wire for excitation of the transducer and transfer of signal to an image processor, and a flexible housing. The rotating transducer is mounted on the tip of the wire and produces a 360° image. Newer mechanical probes that allow mechanical sector plus linear scanning have also been developed (**Table 2**).[4]

BILIARY INTRADUCTAL ULTRASOUND

Traditional noninvasive imaging with US, CT, and magnetic resonance imaging (MRI)/ MRCP are highly sensitive for detection of ductal dilation; however, these imaging modalities are less reliable in determining the etiology, specific location, or extent of disease. Invasive modality such as ERCP and cytologic sampling and/or biopsy is the next step but even after this step, diagnosis remains uncertain in one-third of the patients.[5–7] EUS is a reliable tool in the evaluation of distal biliary system and in contrast to EUS, IDUS provides more reliable evaluation of the proximal biliary system and surrounding structures such as right hepatic artery, portal vein, and the contents of the hepatoduodenal ligament (**Figs. 1** and **2**). The current critical limitations of IDUS are the shallow depth of penetration (<3 cm), and the inability to assess the lymph node involvement and to perform aspiration cytology. The introduction of the IDUS probe in the biliary system is usually by endoscopic or, in rare cases, percutaneous means.[8] The introduction of the small-diameter probe in the bile duct is possible without sphincterotomy in 75% to 80% of patients.[9–11] The newer generation small-diameter probes, which have a monorail design, can be introduced to the biliary system without sphincterotomy over a 0.035-in (0.0889 cm) guide wire.[12] Cannulation

Table 1 Indications for IDUS
Biliary system
Undetected bile duct stone in patients with clinically high suspicion
Indeterminate biliary strictures to aid differentiation between benign and malignant
Local staging and to define longitudinal spread before resection in cholangiocarcinoma
Pancreas
Define pancreatic duct strictures
Intraductal papillary mucinous neoplasms: differentiation between benign and malignant
Neuroendocrine tumors not detected by endoscopic ultrasound
Ampullary adenoma
Local staging: to aid decision for endoscopic resection versus surgical

Table 2
Catheter probe based ultrasound systems (20–30 MHz) for intraductal ultrasound application

	Probe Model	Frequency (MHz)	Working Length (mm)	Probe Diameter (mm)
Fujinon	PL 2226 (20)	20	2200	2.6
	PL 2220 (20)	20	2200	2.0
Olympus	UM-3R	20	2140	2.5
	UM-S20-20R	20	2140	2.0
	UM-S30-20R	30	2140	2.0
	UM-S30-25R	30	2140	2.5
	UM-DP20-25R (dual plane reconstruction)	20	2200	2.5
	UM-BS20-26R-3	20	2140	2.6
	UM-G20-29R (guide wire)	20	2140	2.9

Data from Julia L, Steven C, Ram C, et al. Technology Assessment Committee. Gastrointest Endosc 2006;63:751–4.

of the biliary system can be achieved in nearly 100% of patients without prior sphinc-terotomy with this system.[10] As per the available literature, the time increased for eval-uation of the biliary system with IDUS is only 5 to 10 minutes.[11,13] IDUS is safe, and the reported incidence of pancreatitis is 0.25% in 400 patients.[4] The normal bile duct in an IDUS image has 2 to 3 sonographic layers.[14–16] The resected specimen has been accurately correlated with the initial IDUS interpretation.[17,18] The first sonographic layer is a hypoechoic layer and represents the mucosa, muscularis propria (fibro muscular layer), and fibrous layer of the subserosa. The second sonographic layer is a hyperechoic layer, which is the adipose layer of the subserosa, the serosa, and the interface echo between the serosa and the interface echo between serosa and surrounding organs. If seen, the third layer is a hyperechoic layer and represents an interface echo.[17,18] Sometimes the fibromuscular layer and the perimuscular connec-tive tissue may appear as a single hypoechoic layer, and this limits the ability of IDUS to differentiate T1 and T2 cholangiocarcinoma, although this may not influence the planning of definitive management.

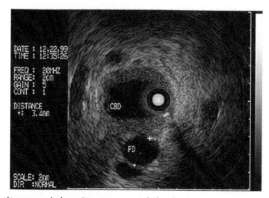

Fig. 1. Intraductal ultrasound showing common bile duct and pancreatic duct.

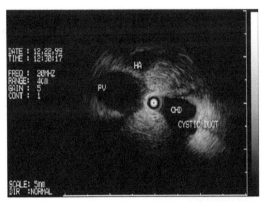

Fig. 2. Intraductal ultrasound showing common hepatic duct, portal vein, and hepatic artery.

Role of Intraductal Ultrasound in Bile Duct Stone Disease

Initial studies suggest a role for IDUS in detecting choledocholithiasis (**Fig. 3**) when the cholangiogram is negative. Palazzo and colleagues prospectively assessed the utility of IDUS in 31 patients with suspected choledocholithiasis. Wire-guided US was used and the bile duct was entered in all patients. The sensitivity of IDUS (97%) was superior to ERCP (81%), fluoroscopy (61%), and US (45%). The missed stone had migrated into the left ductal system and was not detected by IDUS. IDUS is capable of detecting stones less than 5 mm, and effectively differentiates between sludge and air bubbles. There were no reported complications in this study.[19] Another report included 62 patients with suspicion of choledocholithiasis who had cholangiography and IDUS. Confirmation of the stones or sludge was done after sphincterotomy. The accuracy of cholangiography and IDUS was 97%, which was better than cholangiography alone (87%).[20] A study by Tseng and colleagues involving 65 patients with suspected bile

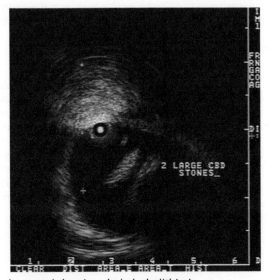

Fig. 3. Intraductal ultrasound showing choledocholithiasis.

duct stones showed that IDUS correctly identified stones in 59 patients. Two false-positive detections were made by IDUS. The overall sensitivity, specificity, and accuracy was 100%, 67%, and 97%, respectively.[21] Another study involving 35 patients to evaluate equivocal findings in cholangiography found that 8 (38%) patients had stones or sludge detected by IDUS.[22] Seven of 8 patients had stones or sludge extracted after sphincterotomy. In contrast, IDUS permitted avoidance of sphincterotomy in 5 patients in whom a suspected stone on cholangiography was shown to be an air bubble by IDUS. Overall, IDUS led to a change in clinical management in 13 patients (37%). The high rate of residual stones and sludge observed in this study compared with previous reports raises questions regarding the quality of the cholangiography, and the clinical significance of the residual stone and sludge is unclear as some of them are small and may pass spontaneously.[23]

A study by Tsuchiya and colleagues, looking at the clinical utility of intraductal ultrasound to decrease early recurrence within 3 years of common bile duct stones after endoscopic papillotomy, suggests that in 14 of 59 patients (23.7%) IDUS detected small residual stones not seen on cholangiography. The recurrence rate was 13.2% (17 of 129 patients) in a historical control group that did not have IDUS versus 3.4% (2 of 59 patients) in the IDUS group ($P<.05$). Multivariate analysis identified non-IDUS status as an independent risk factor for recurrence (odds ratio 5.12, 95% confidence interval [CI] 1.11–23.52, $P = .036$). This study is the only evidence available addressing the utility of IDUS for early recurrence of bile duct stones, but is limited by small sample size and selection of historical controls.[24]

The potential use for IDUS in this patient subgroup is to detect stones in patients who have high suspicion of choledocholithiasis when other imaging modalities have failed to detect them, and to avoid sphincterotomy and its complications in the absence of choledocholithiasis. At the current time, the cost and the relative lack of data limit the use of this technology for this patient subgroup on regular basis.

Role of Intraductal Ultrasound in Bile Duct Strictures

IDUS has a definite role in distinguishing benign and malignant bile duct stricture based on the imaging. The sonographic criteria, which suggest malignancy, include disruption of the normal echo layers, heterogeneity of the internal echo pattern, notching or irregularity of the outer border, papillary surface, or a hypoechoic mass (**Figs. 4 and 5**).[8,10,13,25]

Tamada and colleagues[25] reported an accuracy of 76% for the diagnosis of bile duct cancer in 42 patients. This study did not compare any other imaging modality or histologic confirmation. IDUS was reported to be more accurate in a study by Menzel and colleagues for the diagnosis of bile duct strictures. In all, 56 consecutive patients were studied with wide-ranging pathologies confirmed by histopathology. The underlying pathology included 31 patients with cholangiocarcinoma, gallbladder carcinoma in 5 patients, pancreatic adenocarcinoma in 15 patients, and other benign disorders in 10 patients, including postinflammatory stricture, Caroli disease, choledocholithiasis, and chronic pancreatitis. IDUS was more accurate than EUS in 89% versus 76% ($P<.002$) in determining the nature of the biliary stricture. The T staging (78% vs 54%, $P<.001$) and the determination of resectability (82% vs 76%, $P<.0002$) was accurately determined by IDUS compared with EUS in this study.[13] IDUS was able to differentiate benign strictures after cholecystectomy and Mirrizzi syndrome from invasive cancers. The advantage was more apparent for proximal and mid common bile duct strictures. Experience from the Mayo Clinic suggests similar results: IDUS was more accurate (90%) compared with ERCP and tissue sampling (67%). The sensitivity (54% vs 85%), specificity (87% vs 87%), and accuracy

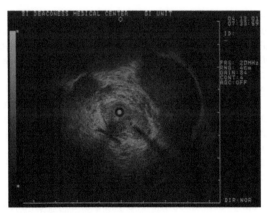

Fig. 4. Intraductal ultrasound in cholangiocarcinoma.

(67% vs 86%) of IDUS was superior to EUS in 21 patients; however, the data did not reach statistical significance. The probe could negotiate the stricture in 26 of the 30 patients (86%), and there were no direct complications related to IDUS in this study.[26] IDUS did not perform well when cholangioscopically directed percutaneous biopsies were obtained. IDUS with percutaneously performed cholangioscopy improved the sensitivity to 100%.[25]

IDUS allows the decision-making in favor of surgery in the absence of histologic confirmation of malignancy by biopsy when there is a disruption of the sonographic wall layer pattern. In the findings of normal sonographic layer pattern by IDUS in a setting of an 8-mm polypoid mass, malignancy is likely and surgery is favored in such a situation. IDUS helps in making decisions about conservative management in the situation of a normal IDUS and cholangiographic abnormality of irregular bile duct. The role of IDUS in primary sclerosing cholangitis (PSC) strictures have not been studied in detail; however, initial data suggest that IDUS may not be of any value in assessing for malignancy in PSC strictures.[27] Tischendorf and colleagues recently reported the value of IDUS for dominant bile duct stenoses in patients with PSC. In their study 40 patients were enrolled and prospectively followed. The patients underwent ERCP and IDUS, as well as tissue sampling. The patients who did not have

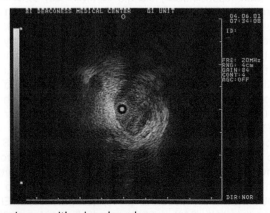

Fig. 5. Cholangiocarcinoma with a lymph node.

positive biopsy or cytology were followed clinically. Eight PSC patients (20%) had dominant bile duct stenoses caused by cholangiocarcinoma, whereas 32 of 40 patients (80%) had benign dominant bile duct stenoses. IDUS was significantly superior to ERCP for detection of malignancy in terms of sensitivity (87.5% vs 62.5%, $P = .05$), specificity (90.6% vs 53.1%, $P<.001$), accuracy (90% vs 55%, $P<.001$), positive predictive value (70% vs 25%, $P<.001$), and negative predictive value (96.7% vs 85%, $P = .049$).[28]

The authors' experience in differentiating benign from malignant biliary stricture in patients who had suspected malignant stricture with negative cytology by IDUS when added to ERCP is very promising, with an accuracy of 92%, sensitivity of 90%, and specificity of 93%. The procedure could not be completed in 2 patients because the stricture could not be traversed with the US probe. The gold standard final diagnosis was based on histopathologic findings or follow-up of at least 12 months.[29] Another study reported on 61 patients with painless jaundice with no mass seen in CT. Forty-three patients had malignant strictures and 18 had benign strictures. ERCP produced 25 false-negative diagnoses, 22 of which were identified as malignant by IDUS. IDUS provided 7 false-negative and 3 false-positive diagnoses. The proportion of patients with malignant strictures who tested positive with IDUS was 2.06 times that of ERCP (95% CI, 1.37–3.10, 83.3% vs 40.5%, $P = .0004$) IDUS increased the accuracy of ERCP from 58% to 90%.[30]

The finding of bile duct thickening by IDUS has been suggested as a marker of a malignant etiology; however, using the same criteria for differentiation between a benign and a malignant lesion is not reliable. This method leads to inaccuracy in T staging in the case of cholangiocarcinoma. One study suggested absence of symmetric wall thickening and protrusion as a marker for inflammatory stricture; however, another study showed poor correlation between wall symmetry and the cause of the biliary stricture.[8,27] A study looked at 45 patients with biliary stricture without mass seen on CT/MRI who underwent ERCP/IDUS. The bile duct thickness by IDUS, less than 7 mm at the stricture site without extrinsic compression, was reported to have a negative predictive value of 100% for excluding malignancy in the study cohort.[31]

There is a definite role for IDUS in defining the longitudinal spread in the case of cholangiocarcinoma. Compared with cholangiography, IDUS accurately defines the longitudinal spread of cholangiocarcinoma toward the liver (84% vs 47%, $P<.05$) and the duodenum (86% vs 43%, $P<.05$).[10] Another study supports the accuracy of proximal extent of the tumor in 92% of the patients.[8]

The current role of IDUS compared with EUS for staging of cholangiocarcinoma is evident in staging the mid duct and bifurcation tumors for accurate T staging. In one study, IDUS was accurate in 77% of patients compared with 54% for staging by EUS.[11] The limited depth of penetration of IDUS precludes assessment of tumor extension outside the hepatoduodenal ligament and lymph node status.[32,33]

As per the available evidence, ERCP/IDUS is a reliable tool in evaluating biliary strictures in the absence of a certain diagnosis with imaging or cytology (**Table 3**). Although ERCP/IDUS has limitations for reliable staging for cholangiocarcinoma, it has an important role in identifying the longitudinal spread for resection planning.

PANCREATIC INTRADUCTAL ULTRASOUND

Suspected pancreatic neoplasm is usually investigated with a CT scan initially, which shows the mass or fullness. Small pancreatic neoplasms are often poorly characterized, and CT fails to detect up to 40% of small pancreatic cancers.[34] In this situation

Table 3
Performance characteristics of ERC/tissue sampling and IDUS in indeterminate bile duct strictures

	Sensitivity	Specificity	Accuracy	PPV	NPV
Vasquez-Seqeiros et al (n = 30 patients): benign 12, malignant 18					
ERCP/tissue sampling	83%	42%	67%	68%	62%
IDUS	89%	92%	90%	94%	85%
Farrell et al[31] (n = 60 patients): benign 29, malignant 31					
ERCP/tissue sampling	48%	100%	73%	100%	64%
IDUS	90%	93%	92%	93%	90%
Stravropoulos et al[32] (n = 43 patients): benign 18, malignant 43					
ERCP/tissue sampling	41%	100%	58%	42%	58%
IDUS	83%	83%	83%	92%	68%

endoscopic procedures are required, namely ERCP, EUS, or for both diagnosis and palliative options. IDUS has been shown to be beneficial for pancreatic diseases.[35–40] Pancreatic sphincterotomy is usually not required for placement of an IDUS probe in the pancreatic duct.[37,41–43] Advancement of the IDUS probe is generally easy in the head and body of the pancreas; however it may be difficult to pass it into the tail of the pancreas. In 153 patients Menzel and colleagues[11] reported insertion of the IDUS catheter in pancreatic head, body, and tail in 94%, 89%, and 55% of patients, respectively. In another study by Furokawa and colleagues,[37] pancreatic cannulation and advancement was possible to the pancreatic head, body, and tail in 100%, 71%, and 35% of the cases. The pancreatic duct is typically seen as single to 3 sonographic layers by an IDUS probe. Three layers are seen with a higher frequency probe of 30 MHz. In 2 studies involving 443 patients, mild pancreatitis was reported in only 4 patients.[11,35]

Role of Intraductal Ultrasound in Pancreatic Duct Strictures

In a study of 25 patients, pancreatic IDUS correctly diagnosed stricture from focal pancreatitis in 23 patients (92%). Two patients were falsely diagnosed to have pancreatic cancer.[35] In another study Furukawa and colleagues compared IDUS to EUS, CT, and endoscopic retrograde pancreatography (ERP) in 26 patients with focal strictures in the pancreatic duct (14 malignant, 12 benign). The sensitivity of IDUS was 100% whereas that of EUS, CT, and ERP was 93%, 64%, and 86%, respectively. The specificity of IDUS was also higher (92% vs 58%, 67%, and 67%, respectively, for EUS, CT, and pancreatography).[36]

Furukawa and colleagues evaluated IDUS in a study of 239 patients with pancreatic disorders, including 48 with adenocarcinoma. IDUS imaged (20 MHz) cystic lesions of less than 30 mm and solid lesions of less than 20 mm in diameter. The entire cross section of the portal, superior mesenteric, and splenic veins were well visualized in all patients. For the diagnosis of pancreatic cancer, the sensitivity of IDUS (100%) was greater than that of EUS (90%), CT (67%), and ERP (90%). The specificity of IDUS (92%) was also higher than that of EUS (60%), CT (67%), and ERP (90%).[35]

Role of Intraductal Ultrasound in Cystic Neoplasm of the Pancreas

IDUS has been shown to be beneficial in the evaluation of cystic neoplasm of the pancreas (**Figs. 6** and **7**).[35,43–45] The data suggest IDUS has higher sensitivity and

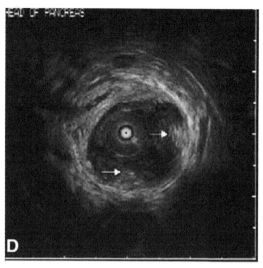

Fig. 6. Intraductal ultrasound picture of intrapapillary mucinous neoplasm.

specificity than EUS. In one study of intraductal papillary mucinous neoplasms (IPMN) of the main pancreatic duct involving 7 patients, IDUS detected abnormal areas that were adenomatous tissue or intraductal carcinoma; however, it failed to differentiate the two. In this same study, IDUS detected a mural nodule in 11 of the 21 patients in side-branch IPMN. The histology confirmed malignancy in 3 patients, adenoma in 7 patients, and hyperplasia in 1 patient. In the 10 patients in whom IDUS did not identify a mural nodule, only 1 was found to have adenoma and the other 9 had hyperplasia. This result suggests that mural nodules seen on IDUS had a high likelihood of a malignancy. Of note, 5 of the 11 mural nodules were not detected with EUS evaluation. IDUS also accurately measures the distance from the main pancreatic duct in the case of a side-branch IPMN, which helps in surgical management.

IDUS was compared with US, CT, EUS, and pancreatoscopy in a study of 31 patients with mucin-producing tumors in whom surgical and histopathologic confirmation was obtained.[42] Six patients had papillary tumors arising within the main

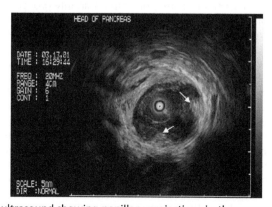

Fig. 7. Intraductal ultrasound showing papillary projections in the pancreatic duct.

duct, and 25 had papillary tumors mainly within cystically dilated branch ducts. Of the 25 patients considered to have side-branch disease, 10 had papillary projections limited to branches and 15 papillary projections had some involvement of the main duct. Evaluation of surgical specimens revealed 8 patients with mucinous cystadeno-carcinoma, 19 with mucinous cystadenoma, and 4 with hyperplasia. Pathology confirmed that all patients with adenocarcinoma had papillary projections in the pancreatic ducts 3 mm or greater in height. The detection rate of such lesions by IDUS (100%) was higher than that for US (29%), CT (21%), EUS (86%), and pancrea-toscopy (83%). Although no patient with hyperplasia had papillary projections of 3 mm or greater, 32% of patients with an adenoma had this finding. Biopsy specimens and cytology specimens obtained at ERCP and pancreatoscopy had a sensitivity and specificity, respectively, of about 60% and 100%. Hara and colleagues reported usefulness of peroral pancreatoscopy (POPS) and IDUS in IPMN for the differentiation of malignant for benign disease. Sixty histopathologically confirmed patients with IPMN underwent POPS or IDUS preoperatively. Lesions protruding 4 mm or more were malignant in 88%. Combination of POPS and IDUS improved the differential diagnosis between benign and malignant IPMN.[43]

These studies demonstrate that IDUS can detect small lesions, and determine the extent of intraductal spread and parenchymal invasion by mucin-producing tumors. This information is useful in determining the necessary extent of resection for mucin-producing tumors involving the main pancreatic duct. Papillary projections, when seen by IDUS, are also helpful in assessing the indication for and required extent of surgery for patients with side-branch disease.

Role of Intraductal Ultrasound in Neuroendocrine Tumors

Initial data suggest that IDUS may improve the evaluation of patients with neuroendo-crine tumors and lead to the identification of tumors arising within the pancreas that have gone unrecognized by other techniques. In one study, IDUS was able to identify the presence of an islet cell tumor in 7 of 7 patients.[39] In one of these patients who had multifocal disease, IDUS accurately determined the number of tumors whereas EUS failed to detect all lesions. The distance from the tumors to the main pancreatic duct was accurately determined, thus aiding preoperative planning of wedge resec-tion, which was possible in 2 patients.

INTRADUCTAL ULTRASOUND FOR AMPULLARY NEOPLASM

Ampullary adenomas are premalignant and in general require endoscopic or surgical resection.[46–48] It is important to define the infiltration of the neoplasm before advising the patient regarding the resection modality, as endoscopic resection has a high recurrence rate. IDUS is the only modality that differentiates sphincter muscle from the remainder of the papilla[49,50] and reliably assesses papillary tumors in terms of size and extent, as well as distinguishing early from advanced tumors (**Fig. 8**).[51,52]

In a prospective study of 27 consecutive patients, 12 had benign tumor and 15 had cancer. IDUS visualized the tumor in 100% of patients, which was better than EUS (59%) and CT (30%). The sensitivity of IDUS was 100% versus 63% for EUS; IDUS had a specificity of 75% versus 50% for EUS. There was also a significant difference in the overall accuracy of tumor diagnosis, which was 89% for IDUS versus 56% for EUS ($P = .05$).[50] In another study of prospective design with 32 patients, the IDUS probe was introduced percutaneously in 24 patients and endoscopically in 8 patients. The accuracy of the IDUS for tumor extent was 88%.[51] A recently published study by Ito and colleagues, involving 40 patients with ampullary neoplasm who underwent

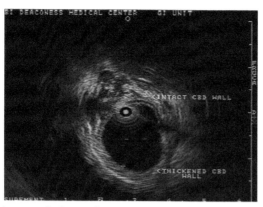

Fig. 8. Intraductal ultrasound of ampullary neoplasm.

resection, surgical (30 patients), and endoscopic (10 patients), reported that 33 patients had adenocarcinoma (14 pT1, 11 pT2, 8 pT3–4) and 7 had adenoma by histology. Tumor detection by EUS and IDUS was achieved in 95% and 100% of the patients, respectively. The diagnostic accuracy of EUS and IDUS in T staging was 62% and 86% in adenoma and pT1, 45% and 64% in pT2, and 88% and 75% in pT3 to 4, respectively. The overall accuracy by EUS and IDUS in T staging was 63% and 78%, respectively ($P = .14$). In 10 patients who underwent endoscopic papillectomy, the accuracy of IDUS in T staging with EUS and IDUS was 80% and 100%, respectively. Ductal infiltration into the biliary duct and the pancreatic duct was correctly assessed in 88% and 90% by EUS, and in both the biliary duct and pancreatic duct in 90% by IDUS. Ductal infiltration was correctly diagnosed by EUS and IDUS in all patients who had a papillectomy.[53] These results suggest that IDUS may be the most accurate imaging modality for the diagnosis and local staging of tumors of the main duodenal papilla, and that patients who undergo endoscopic resection are better staged with IDUS.

SUMMARY

IDUS is an effective tool for imaging in the pancreaticobiliary tree and the adjacent structures for detection of bile duct stones and biliary and pancreatic strictures, assessment of IPMN lesions, and local staging of ampullary neoplasm. IDUS is a complementary examination to ERCP and cholangioscopy as well as EUS.

With the recent addition of the newer cholangioscopic examinations, IDUS will only enhance the ability to diagnose disorders of the pancreaticobiliary tree. The high-resolution intraductal probes that are currently available can assist in evaluation of intraluminal, transmural, and closer extraluminal pathology that may not be adequately seen by fluoroscopy and cholangioscopy/pancreatoscopy. IDUS may be an invaluable tool in evaluating abnormalities in an undilated system, for example, PSC, that is not accessible to cholangioscopy. The high-resolution probes provide exquisite detail of the wall of the pancreaticobiliary tree and the adjacent structures. The same properties that provide the high-resolution imaging limits the depth of penetration and identification of distant structures. In summary, IDUS is a simple, easy to learn, and safe technique that should be considered an integral tool in the therapeutic endoscopist's armamentarium.

REFERENCES

1. Kimmey MB, Martin RW, Silverstein FE. Endoscopic ultrasound probes. Gastroint-est Endosc 1990;36(Suppl 2):S40–6.
2. Martin RW, Silverstein FE, Kimmey MB. A 20 MHz ultrasound system for imaging the intestinal wall. Ultrasound Med Biol 1989;15:273–80.
3. Silverstein FE, Martin RW, Proctor A. Experimental evaluation of an endoscopic ultrasound probe: in vitro and in vivo canine studies. Gastroenterology 1989;96: 1058–62.
4. Levy MJ, Vazquez-Sequeiros E, Wiersema MJ. Evaluation of the pancreatobiliary ductal systems by intraductal US. Gastrointest Endosc 2002;55:397–408.
5. Pugliese V, Conio M, Nicolo G, et al. Endoscopic retrograde forceps biopsy and brush cytology of biliary strictures: a prospective study. Gastrointest Endosc 1995;42:520–6.
6. Schoefl R, Haefner M, Wrba F, et al. Forceps biopsy and brush cytology during endoscopic retrograde cholangiopancreatography for the diagnosis of biliary stenosis. Scand J Gastroenterol 1997;32:363–8.
7. Glasbrenner B, Ardan M, Boeck W, et al. Prospective evaluation of brush cytology of biliary strictures during endoscopic retrograde cholangiopancreatography. Endoscopy 1999;31:712–7.
8. Kuroiwa M, Goto H, Hirooka Y, et al. Intraductal ultrasonography for diagnosis of proximal invasion in extrahepatic bile duct cancer. J Gastroenterol Hepatol 1998; 13:715–9.
9. Noda T, Ido K, Ueno N. Transpapillary intraductal ultrasonography (IDUS) of the bile duct without sphincterotomy. Ultrasound Int 1995;1:141–7.
10. Tamada K, Nagai H, Yasuda Y, et al. Transpapillary intraductal US prior to biliary drainage in the assessment of longitudinal spread of extrahepatic bile duct carci-noma. Gastrointest Endosc 2001;53:300–7.
11. Menzel J, Domschke W. Intraductal ultrasonography (IDUS) of the pancreato-biliary duct system: personal experience and review of the literature. Eur J Ultra-sound 1999;10:105–15.
12. Ascher SM, Evans SR, Goldberg JA, et al. Intraoperative bile duct sonography during laparoscopic cholecystectomy: experience with a 12.5 MHz catheter-based US probe. Radiology 1992;185:493–6.
13. Menzel J, Poremba C, Dietl KH, et al. Preoperative diagnosis of bile duct stric-tures comparison of intraductal ultrasonography with conventional endosonogra-phy. Scand J Gastroenterol 2000;35:77–82.
14. Fujita N, Noda Y, Kobayashi G, et al. Staging of bile duct carcinoma by EUS and IDUS. Endoscopy 1998;30(suppl 1):A132–4.
15. Furukawa T, Naitoh Y, Tsukamoto Y, et al. New technique using intraductal ultra-sound for the diagnosis of diseases of the pancreatobiliary system. J Ultrasound Med 1992;11:607–12.
16. Kuroiwa M, Tsukamoto Y, Naitoh Y, et al. New technique using intraductal ultraso-nography for the diagnosis of bile duct cancer. J Ultrasound Med 1994;13: 189–95.
17. Fujita N, Noda Y, Kobayashi G. Analysis of the layer structure of the gallbladder wall delineated by endoscopic ultrasound using the pinning method. Dig Endosc 1995;7:353–6.
18. Noda Y, Fujita N, Kobayashi G, et al. [Comparison of echograms by a microscan-ner and histological findings of the common bile duct, in vitro study]. Jpn J Gas-troenterol 1997;94:172–9 [in Japanese].

19. Palazzo L. Which test for common bile duct stones? Endoscopic and intraductal ultrasonography. Endoscopy 1997;29:655–65.
20. Das A, Isenberg G, Wong RC, et al. Wire-guided intraductal US: an adjunct to ERCP in the management of bile duct stones. Gastrointest Endosc 2001;54:31.
21. Tseng LJ, Jao YT, Mo LR, et al. Over-the-wire US catheter probe as an adjunct to ERCP in the detection of choledocholithiasis. Gastrointest Endosc 2001;54:720.
22. Catanzaro A, Pfau P, Isenberg GA, et al. Clinical utility of intraductal US for evaluation of choledocholithiasis. Gastrointest Endosc 2003;57:648.
23. Haber GB. Is seeing believing? Gastrointest Endosc 2003;57:712.
24. Tsuchiya S, Tsuyuguchi T, Sakai Y, et al. Clinical utility of intraductal US to decrease early recurrence rate of common bile duct stones after endoscopic papillotomy. J Gastroenterol Hepatol 2008;23:1590–5.
25. Tamada K, Ueno N, Tomiyama T, et al. Characterization of biliary strictures using intraductal ultrasonography: comparison with percutaneous cholangioscopic biopsy. Gastrointest Endosc 1998;47:341–9.
26. Vazquez-Sequeiros E, Baron TH, Clain JE, et al. Evaluation of indeterminate bile duct strictures by intraductal US. Gastrointest Endosc 2002;56:372.
27. Gress F, Chen YK, Sherman S, et al. Experience with a catheter-based ultrasound probe in the bile duct and pancreas. Endoscopy 1995;27:178–84.
28. Tischendorf JJ, Meier PN, Schneider A, et al. Transpapillary intraductal ultrasound in the evaluation of dominant bile duct stenoses in patients with primary sclerosing cholangitis. Scand J Gastroenterol 2007;42:1011–7.
29. Farrell RJ, Agarwal B, Brandwein S, et al. Intraductal US is a useful adjunct to ERCP for distinguishing malignant from benign biliary strictures. Gastrointest Endosc 2002;56:681–7.
30. Stravropoulos S, Larghi A, Verna E, et al. Intraductal ultrasound for the evaluation of patients with biliary strictures and no abdominal mass on computed tomography. Endoscopy 2005;37:715–21.
31. Krishna NB, Saripalli S, Safdar R, et al. Intraductal US in evaluation of biliary strictures without a mass lesion on CT scan or magnetic resonance imaging: significance of focal wall thickening and extrinsic compression at the stricture site. Gastrointest Endosc 2007;66:90–6.
32. Tamada K, Ido K, Ueno N, et al. Assessment of portal vein invasion by bile duct cancer using intraductal ultrasonography. Endoscopy 1995;27:573–8.
33. Tamada K, Kanai N, Tomiyama T, et al. Prediction of the histologic type of bile duct cancer using intraductal US. Abdom Imaging 1999;24:484–90.
34. Palazzo L, Roseau G, Gayet B, et al. Endoscopic ultrasonography in the diagnosis and staging of pancreatic adenocarcinoma. Results of a prospective study with comparison to ultrasonography and CT scan. Endoscopy 1993;25:143–50.
35. Furukawa T, Oohashi K, Yamao K, et al. Intraductal ultrasonography of the pancreas: development and clinical potential. Endoscopy 1997;29:561–9.
36. Furukawa T, Tsukamoto Y, Naitoh Y, et al. Differential diagnosis between benign and malignant localized stenosis of the main pancreatic duct by intraductal ultrasound of the pancreas. Am J Gastroenterol 1994;89:2038–41.
37. Furukawa T, Tsukamoto Y, Naitoh Y, et al. Evaluation of intraductal ultrasonography in the diagnosis of pancreatic cancer. Endoscopy 1993;25:577–81.
38. Inui K, Nakazawa S, Yoshino J, et al. Endoscopy and intraductal ultrasonography. Semin Surg Oncol 1998;15:33–9.
39. Menzel J, Domschke W. Intraductal ultrasonography may localize islet cell tumours negative on endoscopic ultrasound. Scand J Gastroenterol 1998;33:109–12.

40. Menzel J, Foerster EC, Domschke W. Intraductal ultrasound (IDUS) of the pancreas: technique and diagnostic promise. Gut 1992;33:534.
41. Bergman JJ, Rauws EA, Fockens P, et al. Randomized trial of endoscopic balloon dilation versus endoscopic sphincterotomy for removal of bile duct stones. Lancet 1997;349:1124–9.
42. Mukai H, Yasuda K, Nakajima M. Differential diagnosis of mucin-producing tumors of the pancreas by intraductal ultrasonography and peroral pancreato-scopy. Endoscopy 1998;30(suppl 1):A99–A102.
43. Hara T, Yamaguchi T, Ishihara T, et al. Diagnosis and patient management of in-traductal papillary-mucinous tumor of the pancreas by using peroral pancreato-scopy and intraductal ultrasonography. Gastroenterology 2002;122:34–43.
44. Taki T, Goto H, Naitoh Y, et al. Diagnosis of mucin-producing tumor of the pancreas with an intraductal ultrasound system. J Ultrasound Med 1997;16:1–6.
45. Inui K, Nakazawa S, Yoshino J, et al. Mucin-producing tumor of the pancreas—intraluminal ultrasonography. Hepatogastroenterology 1998;45:1996–2000.
46. Rosenberg J, Welch JP, Pyrtek LJ, et al. Benign villous adenomas of the papilla of Vater. Cancer 1986;58:1563–8.
47. Stoke M, Pscherer C. Adenoma-carcinoma sequence in the papilla of Vater. Scand J Gastroenterol 1996;31:376–82.
48. Yamaguchi K, Enjoji M. Carcinoma of the ampulla of Vater: a clinicopathologic study and pathologic staging of 109 cases of carcinoma and 5 cases of adenoma. Cancer 1987;59:506–15.
49. Itoh A, Tsukamoto Y, Naitoh Y, et al. Intraductal ultrasonography for the examina-tion of duodenal papillary region. J Ultrasound Med 1994;13:679–84.
50. Chak A, Isenberg G, Kobayashi K, et al. Prospective evaluation of an over-the-wire catheter US probe. Gastrointest Endosc 2000;51:202–5.
51. Itoh A, Goto H, Naitoh Y, et al. Intraductal ultrasonography in diagnosing tumor extension of cancer of the papilla of Vater. Gastrointest Endosc 1997;45:251–60.
52. Menzel J, Hoepffher N, Sulkowski U, et al. Polypoid tumors of the major duodenal papilla: preoperative staging with intraductal US, EUS, and CT—a prospective, histopathologically controlled study. Gastrointest Endosc 1999;49:349–57.
53. Ito K, Fujita N, Noda Y, et al. Preoperative evaluation of ampullary neoplasm with EUS and transpapillary intraductal US: a prospective and histopathologically controlled study. Gastrointest Endosc 2007;66:740–7.

Confocal Endomicroscopy

Alexander Meining, MD

KEYWORDS

- Bile duct • Confocal • Endomicroscopy
- Endoscopy • Imaging

Biliary strictures can be caused by various inflammatory and neoplastic diseases, both benign and malignant.[1,2] To ensure the best outcome for patients presenting with biliary strictures, an accurate and rapid diagnosis is critical. However, the differentiation between malignant and benign biliary strictures remains challenging, even with the use of endoscopic retrograde cholangiography (ERC).[3,4]

Therefore ERC, which provides direct access to the bile duct, is usually performed in conjunction with tissue sampling of a biliary stricture. Previous methods, however, revealed only poor sensitivity and low negative predictive value of biliary biopsies or brush cytology.[5–8] Hence, there is a need to improve diagnostic accuracy for the differentiation of biliopancreatic strictures.

CONFOCAL LASER ENDOMICROSCOPY

The use of a confocal microscope enables nonsuperficial microscopic imaging of untreated tissue without previous fixation and preparation of slices. The technical principle is to have focused light passed through a confocal aperture, thereby reducing scattered light above and below the plane. However, only one single spot, called confocal, can be imaged at once. To overcome this and to have dynamic images, all light spots have to be scanned in the horizontal (and vertical) plane.

Applied to biologic tissue, these same technical elements enable microscopic imaging tissue. Inoue and colleagues were the first to evaluate such a technology ex vivo with fresh biopsy specimens of the human intestine.[9] These first data demonstrated that it is possible to visualize cellular structures in untreated tissue. Certain contrasting features of malignant mucosa that differed from benign mucosa could be identified, although the overall quality and image resolution was poor.

The author is a copatent holder on CholangioFlex probes. Equipment has been supplied by Mauna Kea Technologies (Paris, France) for conducting clinical studies on pCLE with various indications.
Department of Medicine II, Klinikum rechts der Isar, Technical University of Munich, Ismaningerstr. 22, 81675 Munich, Germany
E-mail address: alexander.meining@lrz.tum.de

giendo.theclinics.com

Since these early ex vivo feasibility studies, the greatest challenge of confocal fluorescence microscopy has been the miniaturization of the system, to incorporate it into standard endoscopy equipment. Today there are mainly 2 options available, based on the high-level architecture of the laser scanning system, which can be either proximal or distal to the laser light transmission: a tip-integrated confocal laser endomicroscope and a flexible fiber-based confocal miniprobe.

The tip-based system integrates a confocal endomicroscope in the distal tip of a conventional colonoscope (a joint venture between Pentax, Japan and Optiscan, Australia). A single optical fiber acts as both the illumination point source and detection pinhole. This situation means that white-light endoscopy and confocal endomicroscopy are performed simultaneously, but displayed sequentially on the monitor display. The endoscope has a regular working channel and water-cleansing channel. The diameter of both the distal tip and the insertion tube is 12.8 mm, making the device essentially suitable for colonoscopy or gastroscopy but not for smaller lumens such as in the biliary or pancreatic ducts. The tip of the endomicroscope is also rigid along several centimeters, making it less maneuverable than a standard endoscope.

Another device has been introduced as a flexible probe-based confocal laser endomicroscopy (pCLE) system (Cellvizio, Mauna Kea Technologies, France). Here, both the laser scanning unit and light source are outside the body of the patient, making the confocal miniprobe a "passive" device. The laser beam (488 nm) is transported via confocal miniprobes and is sequentially scanned through each one of the tens of thousands of optical fibers bundled together and terminated by a distal micro-objective. The miniprobes are very flexible, and diameters range from 0.9 mm to 2.5 mm. Thereby, this probe-based system may easily be introduced through the working channels of endoscopes, including small-caliber cholangioscopes. Confocal endomicroscopy image data are collected at a frame rate of 12 frames per second, enabling video quality. The field of view ranges from a 240-μm diameter field to a 600-μm diameter field, depending on which specific probe is used. Smallest lateral and axial resolutions are 1 μm and 3 μm, respectively. Miniprobes are reusable several times, and the whole setup (probes connected to laser scanning unit and personal computer with dedicated acquisition and editing/quantification software) can easily be transported in the endoscopy suite (**Fig. 1**).

When using any of the confocal laser endomicroscopy systems, the application of a fluorophore is mandatory for mucosal fluorescence imaging. Topically applied agents such as cresyl violet,[10] acriflavine,[11] or fluorescein[12] have been evaluated. However, the use of these dyes seems inappropriate if a continuous water flow is necessary, such as in the bile and pancreatic ducts during cholangioscopy. Alternatively, endomicroscopic images can be acquired after intravenous application of fluorescein.[6,13] This approach has the further benefit that blood vessels become clearly visible.[14,15] Moreover, because angiogenesis has been suggested as an essential step in the development of cancers, documentation of blood flow, vessel density, and configuration is especially relevant.[16]

DEVELOPMENT OF pCLE FOR BILIARY IMAGING

Taking into consideration the shortcomings in the differential diagnosis of biliary strictures and the potentials of pCLE for in vivo histopathology, it became evident that this new diagnostic modality might be a useful adjunct for improvement of diagnostic accuracy. Nevertheless, several challenges had to be tackled. New probes had to be designed that would be flexible and small enough to be introduced even via small

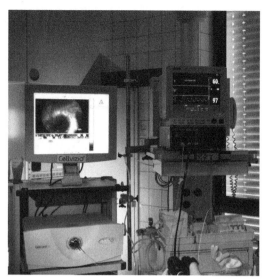

Fig. 1. Portable probe-based system for confocal laser scanning endomicroscopy (Cellvizio, Mauna Kea Technologies, France). The confocal miniprobe is connected to a laser scanning unit, which itself is connected to a standard computer. The whole setup can easily be moved.

instrumentation channels, but rigid enough to enable exact placement and maneuverability of the probe tip.

Conventional miniprobes that have been previously used with success in the upper and lower gastrointestinal tract[17,18] were applied initially. Albeit small enough for introduction into the common bile duct directly via a duodenoscope, the probes were too rigid to be oriented and pushed through the papilla's orifice. Intraductal placement was only possible via 11.5F guiding catheters but even then the procedure was troublesome, and further evaluation of a stricture was difficult by solely fluoroscopic guidance. The tip of the probe, which is radio-opaque, was used as a marker of the position of the probe in the duct. The images were not reliable, due to the impaired maneuverability of the probe and the often-occurring inability to place the probe tip onto the mucosa. Because the pCLE image is generated in a prograde fashion, the tip should ideally be placed in a perpendicular angle to the tissue, or at least tangential rather than in a longitudinal manner. This placement is difficult in small ducts due to conformational constraints. In addition, the probe tends to glide into the stricture's lumen, so imaging of its borders is almost impossible. Further miniaturization of probes with the potential to place the tip under direct visual guidance was therefore mandatory. A major breakthrough was achieved by creating a probe with a diameter below 1 mm for insertion into the instrumentation channel of cholangioscopes (**Fig. 2**) or standard endoscopic retrograde cholangiopancreatography (ERCP) catheters. Reduction of the number of fibers in the optical bundle and a dedicated coating of the probe finally enabled sufficient stiffness for introduction and maneuverability of the probe. The only shortcoming was that, due to the reduction in the number of fibers, the field of view had to be reduced to a diameter of 325 μm, nevertheless still enabling sufficient imaging. The minimum lateral resolution achievable with such miniaturized probes was 3.5 μm. Based on several prototype trials, and according to data acquired in pig models and in anatomic analysis of resected biliary human epithelium, the confocal imaging depth was set to 40 to 70 μm. This specially designed

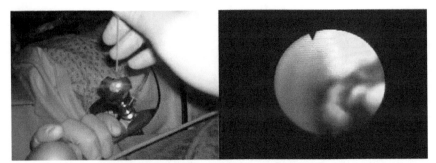

Fig. 2. CholangioFlex probe (diameter: 0.9 mm) being introduced into the instrumentation channel of a cholangioscope (Karl Storz, Germany) (*left*) and cholangioscopic view of miniprobe attached onto the biliary epithelium (*right*).

miniprobe—the so-called CholangioFlex (Mauna Kea Technologies, Paris, France)—is now Food and Drug Administration (FDA)-cleared, Conformité Européene (CE)-marked, and commercially available.

ENDOMICROSCOPIC HALLMARKS FOR MALIGNANCY

After it became possible to perform pCLE in the bile duct under visual guidance via cholangioscopes, certain hallmarks had to be identified for further differentiation of benign versus malignant epithelium. The author's group conducted a feasibility study of further differentiation of biliary strictures by pCLE via peroral cholangioscopy.[19] A total of 14 patients with biliary strictures were examined, 8 of which were of benign and 6 of malignant origin. All strictures could be reached with the CholangioFlex probe. In general, 2 different patterns could be identified.

The first specific pattern was found predominately in patients with cancers, and was characterized by a dark-gray background without identification of specific mucosal structures, but large white streaks resembling fluorescein-filled tortuous, dilated, and saccular vessels with inconsistent branching. In the dynamic video sequences, erythrocytes could easily be identified rushing through these "streaks," demonstrating that indeed, vascular structures could be identified (**Fig. 3**).

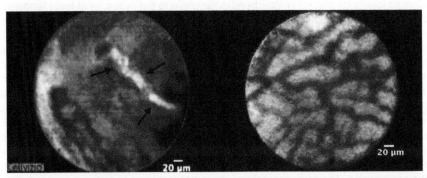

Fig. 3. pCLE images of benign and malignant biliary epithelium. Neoplastic epithelium (*left*) is characterized by black areas with decreased uptake of fluorescein, irregular epithelium, and irregular vessels (*arrows*), whereas regular epithelium is determined by a fine netlike reticular pattern (*right*).

The second pattern, associated with benign strictures and normal tissue, comprised a fine, netlike, reticular pattern of different gray scales or small dark-gray and thin villous structures, but no "white streaks." Applying these hallmarks as defined, sensitivity, specificity, and overall diagnostic accuracy for detection of neoplasia was 5 of 6 (83%), 7 of 8 (88%), and 12 of 14 (86%), respectively. Furthermore, sensitivity could be considerably improved from 50% to 83% if confocal miniprobes were used instead of solely standard histopathology. It was therefore concluded that pCLE might be an ideal adjunct to cholangioscopy for further characterization of visible lesions and masses.

Meanwhile, the author's group and others have been able to further increase their experience. Based on their previous and current data, the following hallmarks for malignancy in the biliary tract are proposed:

- Loss of reticular pattern of epithelial bands of less than 20 μm
- Detection of irregular epithelial lining, villi, or glandlike structure
- Tortuous, dilated, and saccular vessels with inconsistent branching
- Presence of "black areas" of more than 60 to 80 μm (focally decreased uptake of fluorescein)

Further approaches of pCLE via cholangioscopes have meanwhile been tested. The author's group was able to detect and further differentiate pancreatic strictures such as intraductal papillary mucinous neoplasms (IPMNs).[20] In this study, a villous structure of the mucosa resembling an IPMN of the oncocytic type was easily identified. In these cases, pCLE might help to further clarify localization and types of IPMN for a more targeted surgical resection.

CURRENT LIMITATIONS AND OUTLOOK

Current data on pCLE in the biliaropancreatic system are promising but still sparse, taking into consideration that CholangioFlex probes were launched in May 2008. Hence, everyone with an interest in this new method (including the author himself) is still in his or her learning phase. The pCLE hallmarks for further malignancy seem to be reliable, particularly in comparison with standard tissue sampling methods; nevertheless, it has to be borne in mind that these hallmarks are based on a fairly low number of patients. In addition, it has not been clarified how accurate pCLE can be for further differentiation of inflammation from malignancy. Moreover, so far there are only case reports on pCLE for pancreatic imaging. For this reason a multicenter registry has been initiated, including longitudinal follow-up, to further test the accuracy of proposed hallmarks of pCLE and perhaps identify new criteria for malignancy versus inflammation. Other indications could be the use of pCLE for the monitoring of mucosal alterations during photodynamic therapy, assessment of vessel density during ongoing chemotherapy, or a combination of the method with other imaging modalities to further increase diagnostic accuracy.

Furthermore, it remains unclear whether it is necessary to perform pCLE via cholangioscopes or whether positioning of the probes via standard ERCP catheters under fluoroscopic control is equally effective. The cholangioscopic approach might be more precise, but it has to be borne in mind that the procedure requires 2 investigators. Use of the probe in conjunction with the SpyGlass system (Boston Scientific, USA) by a single investigator is very demanding because a single person has to control the duodenoscope, the cholangioscope, and the confocal miniprobe. Last but not least, the cost-effectiveness of pCLE should be assessed in comparison with other methods, including new cytologic methods that also show promising results for detecting malignancy, such as the fluorescence in situ hybridization technique.[21]

REFERENCES

1. Anderson CD, Pinson CW, Berlin J, et al. Diagnosis and treatment of cholangiocarcinoma. Oncologist 2004;9:43–57.
2. Jarnagin WR, Shoup M. Surgical management of cholangiocarcinoma. Semin Liver Dis 2004;24:189–99.
3. Uhlmann D, Wiedmann M, Schmidt F, et al. Management and outcome in patients with Klatskin-mimicking lesions of the biliary tree. J Gastrointest Surg 2006;10:1144–50.
4. Rösch T, Hofrichter K, Frimberger E, et al. ERCP or EUS for tissue diagnosis of biliary strictures? A prospective comparative study. Gastrointest Endosc 2004;60:390–6.
5. Weber A, von Weyhern C, Fend F, et al. Endoscopic transpapillary brush cytology and forceps biopsy in patients with hilar cholangiocarcinoma. World J Gastroenterol 2008;14:1097–101.
6. Elek G, Gyökeres T, Schäfer E, et al. Early diagnosis of pancreatobiliary duct malignancies by brush cytology and biopsy. Pathol Oncol Res 2005;11:145–55.
7. Fogel EL, deBellis M, McHenry L, et al. Effectiveness of a new long cytology brush in the evaluation of malignant biliary obstruction: a prospective study. Gastrointest Endosc 2006;63:71–7.
8. Patel T, Singh P. Cholangiocarcinoma: emerging approaches to a challenging cancer. Curr Opin Gastroenterol 2007;23:317–23.
9. Inoue H, Igari T, Nishikage T, et al. A novel method of virtual histopathology using laser-scanning confocal microscopy in-vitro with untreated fresh specimens from the gastrointestinal mucosa. Endoscopy 2000;32:439–43.
10. George M, Meining A. Cresyl violet as a fluorophore for future in vivo histopathology. Endoscopy 2003;35:585–90.
11. Kiesslich R, Goetz M, Burg J, et al. Diagnosing *Helicobacter pylori* in vivo by confocal laser endoscopy. Gastroenterol 2005;128:2119–23.
12. Polglase AL, McLaren WJ, Skinner SA, et al. A fluorescence confocal endomicroscope for in vivo microscopy of the upper- and the lower-GI tract. Gastrointest Endosc 2005;62:686–95.
13. Becker V, Vercauteren T, Hann von Weyhern C, et al. High resolution miniprobe-based confocal microscopy in combination with video mosaicing. Gastrointest Endosc 2007;66:1001–7.
14. von Delius S, Feussner H, Wilhelm D, et al. Transgastric in-vivo histopathology in the peritoneal cavity by miniprobe based confocal fluorescence microscopy in a porcine model. Endoscopy 2007;39:407–11.
15. Meining A, Wallace MB. Endoscopic imaging of angiogenesis in vivo. Gastroenterol 2008;134:915–8.
16. Hicklin DJ, Ellis LM. Role of the vascular endothelial growth factor pathway in tumor growth and angiogenesis. J Clin Oncol 2005;23:1011–27.
17. Meining A, Saur D, Bajbouj M, et al. In-vivo histopathology for detection of gastrointestinal neoplasia using a portable, confocal miniprobe—an examiner blinded analysis. Clin Gastroenterol Hepatol 2007;5:1261–7.
18. Becker V, von Delius S, Bajbouj M, et al. Intravenous application of fluorescein for confocal laser scanning microscopy: evaluation of contrast dynamics and image

quality with increasing injection-to-imaging time. Gastrointest Endosc 2008;68: 319–23.

19. Meining A, Frimberger E, Becker V, et al. Detection of cholangiocarcinoma in vivo using miniprobe-based confocal fluorescence microscopy. Clin Gastroenterol Hepatol 2008;6:1057–60.

20. Meining A, Phillip V, Gaa J, et al. Pancreaticoscopy with miniprobe-based confocal laserscanning-microscopy of an intraductal papillary mucinous neoplasm. Gastrointest Endosc 2009;69:1178–80.

21. Levy MJ, Baron TH, Clayton AC, et al. Prospective evaluation of advanced molecular markers and imaging techniques in patients with indeterminate bile duct strictures. Am J Gastroenterol 2008;103:1263–73.

Optical Coherence Tomography for Bile and Pancreatic Duct Imaging

Pier Alberto Testoni, MD[a],*, Benedetto Mangiavillano, MD[b]

KEYWORDS

- Optical coherence tomography • Common bile duct
- Main pancreatic duct • Sphincter of Oddi • OCT
- Pancreatobiliary system • GI tract • Gut • Ex-vivo • In-vivo

Optical coherence tomography (OCT) is an optical imaging modality introduced in 1991[1] that performs high-resolution, cross-sectional, subsurface tomographic imaging of the microstructure in materials and biologic systems by measuring back-scattered or back-reflected infrared light. OCT has been used for biomedical applications where many factors affect the feasibility and effectiveness of any imaging technique. The highly scattering and absorbing living tissues greatly limit the application of optical imaging modalities.

In the last decade, OCT technology has evolved from an experimental laboratory tool to a new diagnostic imaging modality with a wide spectrum of clinical applications in medical practice, including the gastrointestinal (GI) tract and pancreaticobiliary ductal system.

In vitro studies demonstrated the feasibility of OCT in the GI tract and its capability to visualize the mucosa and submucosa of the gut;[2] the muscular-layer structure has also been recognized in a study.[3]

Subsequent studies were, therefore, performed in ex vivo tissue specimens and aimed at comparing OCT imaging with histology, to assess the reliability of the OCT technique to identify and recognize the GI and pancreaticobiliary wall structure. OCT was shown to clearly recognize and differentiate the layer structure of the wall.[4]

In vivo studies confirmed the possibility of OCT to recognize the multiple-layer structure of the GI wall. In these studies, the GI tract wall was identified as a multiple layer structure characterized by a sequence of hyper- and hyporeflective layers, with a variable homogenicity of the backscattered signal.[5] Neoplastic and non-neoplastic

[a] Division of Gastroenterology and Gastrointestinal Endoscopy, Vita-Salute San Raffaele University, Scientific Institute San Raffaele Hospital, Via Olgettina 60, 20132 Milan, Italy
[b] Department of Gastroenterology and Gastrointestinal Endoscopy, San Paolo University Hospital, Via A. di Rudinì 8, 20142 Milan, Italy
* Corresponding author.
E-mail address: testoni.pieralberto@hsr.it (P.A. Testoni).

Gastrointest Endoscopy Clin N Am 19 (2009) 637–653
doi:10.1016/j.giec.2009.06.006
1052-5157/09/$ – see front matter © 2009 Elsevier Inc. All rights reserved.

tissue also showed different light backscattering patterns.[6–8] In addition, a relevant characteristic of this technique is the capability of visualizing microscopic structures, such as villi, blood vessels, lymphoid aggregates, crypts and submucosal glands.[9] When the probe is lightly placed on the ductal surface, the depth of penetration is mainly limited to the superficial layers; the superficial epithelium, lamina propria, and the upper part of submucosa are clearly visualized. When the probe is placed firmly against the mucosal surface, submucosa and muscularis propria can be clearly visualized, but details of the superficial layers of the mucosa are lost. Based on these features, OCT could find clinical utility in the recognition of epithelial dysplasia and early detection of cancer.[10,11]

The possibility to introduce the OCT probe into a standard transparent catheter for cannulation during an endoscopic retrograde cholangiopancreatography (ERCP) procedure also allows investigation of the epithelial layers of the pancreatobiliary ductal system and sphincter of Oddi (SO). Despite the recent introduction of the intraductal ultrasound, OCT presents a resolution of 10- to 25-fold better. Therefore, this device is an attractive imaging technique to study the pancreatobiliary ductal system, considering also the technical difficulties to gain a target biliary or pancreatic biopsy, and the low-diagnostic sensitivity of the brush cytology. Moreover, OCT allows an in vivo diagnosis of the pancreatic and biliary ductal system during ERCP.[12]

OPTICAL COHERENCE TOMOGRAPHY PHYSICAL PRINCIPLE

The physical principle of OCT is similar to that of B-mode ultrasound imaging, except that the intensity of infrared light, rather than sound waves, is measured. Ultrasound imaging is accomplished by measuring the delay time (echo delay) for an incidental ultrasonic pulse to be reflected back from structures within tissue. The velocity of the sound is slow, relative to the light; therefore, the echo delay time can be measured electronically. OCT measurements of the delay time cannot be performed easily using standard electronic detection because the velocity of the light is 10^6 times greater than the sound. Therefore, a technique known as low coherence interferometry (LCI) is used to measure the delay time of reflected light from within tissue.[13]

LCI functions by comparing light reflected from internal microstructures in the tissue specimen to light traversing a reference path of known path length. Infrared light generated from the low coherence source is split evenly, half to the sample and half toward a moving mirror. Light is reflected off the references mirror and from within the sample and recombined in the beam splitter (50/50). If the light reflected from within the sample travels is the same distance (optical) as light from the reference mirror, interference will occur at the detector. OCT measures the intensity of this interference, which represents the intensity of back reflection. Moving the mirror changes the distance traveled by light in the reference arm, allowing back-reflecting intensity to be assessed at different depths within the tissue. The back-reflecting intensity is plotted as a function of depth analogous to conventional ultrasound imaging. The shaded area represents the portion of the system that would be present within the endoscope, consisting primarily of an optical fiber, lens, and a mirror.

More specifically, interference will occur if the two path lengths are matched to within the property of light, known as the coherence length, which is analogous to the pulse duration. The magnitude of the interference, proportional to the reflected or backscattered light from structures inside tissue, is then plotted as a function of depth in a manner similar to A-mode ultrasound. A cross-sectional image is created by acquiring multiple axial scans as the beam position is scanned across the sample.

The resulting data are displayed as a gray scale or false color images. The image contrast in an OCT image arises from variation in the optical reflectance of the tissue.

OCT devices use a low-power infrared light with a wavelength ranging from 750 to 1300 nm in which the only limiting factor is the scattering of light. OCT images are then generated from measuring the echo time delay and the intensity of backscattered light.[14,15] Wavelengths of the infrared light used in OCT are one to two orders of magnitude higher than ultrasound wavelength, so OCT technology can yield a lateral and axial spatial resolution of approximately10 micron, which is 10- to 25-fold better than that of available high-frequency ultrasound imaging.[16] The spatial resolution of OCT images is nearly equivalent to that of histologic sections. The depth of penetration of OCT imaging is approximately from 1 to 3 mm, depending upon tissue structure, depth of focus of the probe used, and pressure applied to the tissue surface. Although the progressive increase in ultrasound resolution is accompanied by a corresponding decrease in depth of penetration, a similar trade-off between resolution and depth of penetration does not occur in OCT imaging.

Three types of scanning patterns are available for OCT imaging: radial,[17,18] longitudinal,[19,20] and transverse (**Fig. 1**).[21] The radial-scan probe directs the OCT beam radially, giving images that are displayed in a circular, radar like plot. Radial scanning can easily image large areas of tissue by moving the probe over the tissue surface. It has the highest definition when the probe is inserted within a small diameter lumen; the OCT images become progressively coarser when a large-diameter lumen is scanned, which is caused by the progressive increase of pixel spacing with the increase in distance between the probe and the tissue. The linear and transverse probes scan the longitudinal and transverse positions of the OCT beam at a fixed angle, generating rectangular images of longitudinal and transverse planes at a given angle with respect to the probe. The advantage of linear scanning is that the pixel spacing in the transverse direction is uniform and can better image a definite area of the scanned tissue, especially in the presence of large-diameter and noncircular lumens, in which maintaining constant distance from the probe to the surface over the entire circumferential scan may be impossible. Transverse scanning modality provides a better depth of

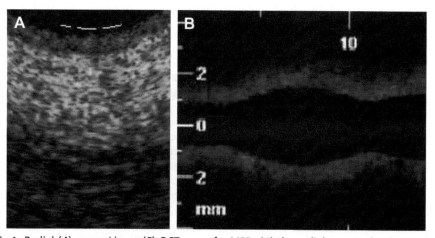

Fig. 1. Radial (*A*) versus Linear (*B*) OCT scan of a MPD. (*A*) the radial-scan probe directs the OCT beam radially, giving images that are displayed in a circular, radar like plot. (*B*) the linear probe scans the longitudinal positions of the OCT beam at a fixed angle, generating rectangular images of longitudinal planes at a given angle with respect to the probe.

field. Depth of field is the range of distances from the probe over which optimal resolution of scanning can be obtained; current OCT scans permit imaging depths of up to 2 to 3 mm in tissues, by using probes with different focuses.

OPTICAL COHERENCE TOMOGRAPHY TECHNIQUE FOR PANCREATICOBILIARY DUCTAL SYSTEM IMAGING

OCT imaging of the pancreaticobiliary ductal system can be done in humans by using narrow-diameter, catheter-based probes. The catheter-based probe has a diameter of 1.2 mm and consists of a rotating OCT probe encased in a transparent outer sheath, which remains stationary while the rotating probe has a pull-back movement of 1 mm/s, with an acquisition rate of 10 frames per second. By this technique a segment of tissue 5.5 cm long can be filmed over a 55-second period (**Fig. 2**). On the tip of the probe is placed a radiopaque marker, allowing the operator to have the correct position of the probe inside the duct during ERCP and to visualize the correct site of the duct from which the pull-back maneuver starts. Infrared light is delivered to the imaging site through a single optical fiber .006″ in diameter.

A near-focus OCT probe (Pentax - Lightlab Imaging, Westford, MA, USA) is available with a penetration depth of 1 mm, resolution approximately 10 μm, and outer diameter 1.2 mm. The probe operates at 1.2 to 1.4 μm center wavelength (nominal value 1.3 μm), with scan frequency ranging from 1000 to 4000 kHz (nominal value 3125 kHz); radial and longitudinal scanning resolutions have an operating range in tissue of 15 to 20 μm (nominal value 18 μm) and 21 to 27 μm (nominal value 24 μm), respectively. The probe can be inserted through the accessory channel of the side-view endoscope, inside a standard transparent ERCP catheter (**Fig. 3**). The ERCP catheter allows protection of the thin and fragile OCT probe, because the elevator of the side-view endoscope could be traumatic during the probe insertion into the ductal system. The pull-back technique is the standard technique used for the study of the pancreaticobiliary system. OCT scanning can be done either by keeping the OCT probe in the ERCP catheter or leaving it in the duct outside the catheter. Although the transparent surface of the ERCP catheter makes it difficult to examine the inner layer corresponding to the ductal epithelium, the diagnostic capacity of OCT is not substantially affected by the catheter sheath comparing with images obtained keeping the probe outside the catheter (**Fig. 4**).

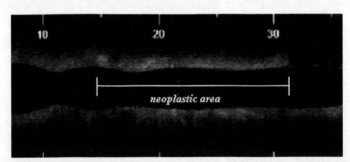

Fig. 2. OCT longitudinal image of the MPD wall obtained by the pull-back technique. The MPD wall structures close to the ductal lumen and the margin between the tumor-involved and tumor-free MPD segments are clearly recognizable from the difference in light back-scattering (hyporeflective as a whole in the non-neoplastic segment, hyper-reflective in the neoplastic segment).

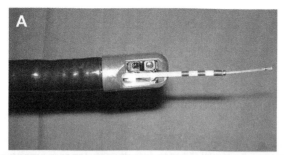

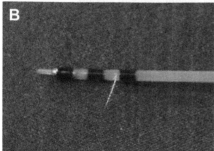
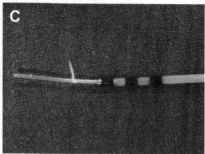

Fig. 3. OCT probe protected by the ERCP catheter inside of the operative channel of the side view endoscope (*A*). OCT working probe inside (*B*) and outside (*C*) the ERCP catheter; the visible red laser is the infrared light given out from the tip of the probe.

From a clinical point of view, OCT imaging of the pancreatic and biliary ductal system could improve the diagnostic accuracy for ductal epithelial changes and the differential diagnosis between neoplastic and non-neoplastic lesions, because in several conditions X-ray morphology obtained by ERCP and other imaging techniques may be nondiagnostic, and the sensitivity of intraductal brush cytology during ERCP procedures is highly variable.

OPTICAL COHERENCE TOMOGRAPHY RECOGNITION OF THE PANCREATICOBILIARY WALL STRUCTURE IN NORMAL CONDITIONS

To date, visualization of the epithelium of the main pancreatic duct (MPD) has been obtained mainly post mortem[22] and ex vivo in humans,[23] while in vivo from one study in animals[24] and another in humans.[12] Normal biliary ductal system has been investigated in humans, ex vivo in a study[4] and in vivo, in two ERCP-based studies.[25,26] SO structure has also been investigated in normal and pathological conditions either in ex vivo or in vivo studies.[4,27]

In a recent study by our group,[4] OCT imaging of MPD, common bile duct (CBD) and SO normal structure has been shown to be able to provide features that were similar to those observed in the corresponding histologic specimens in 80% of sections; the agreement between OCT and histology in the definition of normal wall was good (81.8%). OCT images identified three differentiated layers up to a depth of about 1 mm. From the surface of the duct, it was possible to recognize an inner hyporeflective layer corresponding to the single layer of epithelial cells close to the lumen, an intermediate homogeneous hyper-reflective layer corresponding to the fibro-muscular layer surrounding the epithelium, and an outer, less definite, hyporeflective layer corresponding to the smooth muscular structure within a connective tissue in the CBD

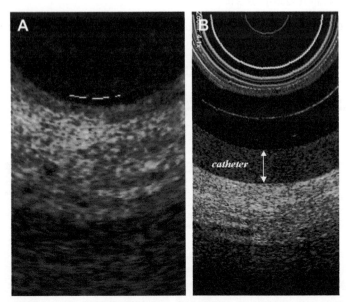

Fig. 4. Magnification of an OCT image from the MPD wall stricture in EUS documented normal pancreas, with OCT probe outside (*A*) and inside (*B*) the ERCP catheter. (*A*) A well-defined three-layer architecture is visible, with a superficial hyporeflective band corresponding to the single layer of epithelial cells surrounding the MPD, an intermediate hyperreflective layer corresponding to the connective-fibro-muscular layer surrounding the epithelium, and an outer hypo-reflective layer corresponding to the connective and acinar structure close to the ductal wall epithelium. (*B*) The inner hyporeflective layer is compressed by the ERCP catheter sheet (*white arrow*) and is not visible; however, the layer structure and homogeneous back-scattering of the signal are maintained.

and at the level of the SO, and connective-acinar structure in the main pancreatic duct (**Figs. 5–7**).

Based on our studies, the inner, hyporeflective layer shows a mean thickness of 0.05 mm (range: 0.04–0.08 mm) and a homogeneous back-scattering of the signal in all the imaged sites; thickness, surface, regularity, and reflectance degree of this layer does not substantially differ in the CBD, MPD and SO. The intermediate layer shows a mean thickness of 0.41 mm (range: 0.34–0.48 mm) in the CBD, 0.42 mm (range: 0.36–0.56 mm) in the MPD and 0.29 mm (range 0.23–0.37 mm) in the SO. The layer thickness is substantially similar in the MPD and in CBD, while appeared reduced by 25% at level of the SO. The layer appears hyper-reflective when compared with the inner and outer layers and the reflectance degree does not change in all of the imaged sites. The outer layer appears recognizable until a depth of 1 mm from the lumen and is hyporeflective in all the imaged sites. Multiple, hyper-reflective, longitudinal strips are recognizable at level of the CBD and the SO. These longitudinal strips are more pronounced and hyper-reflective in the SO, so the layer appeared at this level is less hyporeflective than in the CBD.

The three layers show a linear, regular surface and each layer had a homogeneous back-scattered signal in every frame; however, the differentiation between the intermediate and outer layer appears more difficult than between the inner and intermediate layer. The thickness of the inner and intermediate layers measured by OCT is similar to those measured by histology; the muscular and connective-acinar structure

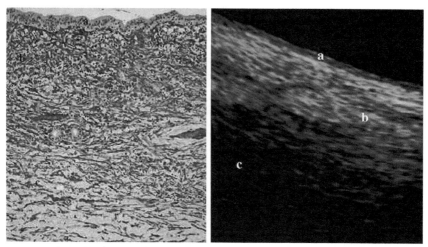

Fig. 5. Magnification of an OCT image from the normal CBD wall, confirmed by histology. From the surface of the duct, up to a depth of 1 mm, the following layers are recognizable: (a) the single layer of epithelial cells, approximately 0.04 to 0.06 mm thick, visible as a superficial, hyporeflective band; (b) the connective-muscular layer surrounding the epithelium, visible as a hyper-reflective layer approximately 0.34 to 0.48 mm thick; and (c) the connective layer visible as a hyporeflective layer with longitudinal hyper-reflective strips (smooth muscle fibers).

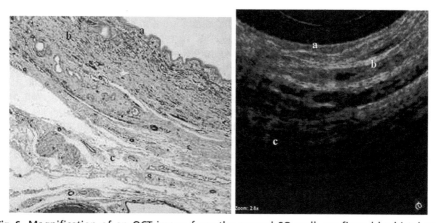

Fig. 6. Magnification of an OCT image from the normal SO wall, confirmed by histology. From the surface of the duct, up to a depth of 1 mm, the following layers are recognizable: (a) the single layer of epithelial cells, approximately 0.04 to 0.08 mm thick, visible as a superficial, hyporeflective band; (b) the connective-muscular layer surrounding the epithelium, visible as a hyper-reflective layer approximately 0.23 to 0.37 mm thick; and (c) the connective layer visible as a hyporeflective layer with longitudinal relatively hyper-reflective strips (smooth muscle fibers).Within, the intermediate and outer layer vessels are also recognizable visualized as nonreflecting areas surrounded by a hyporeflective endothelium. Margins between the intermediate and outer layer are poorly recognizable because of the irregular distribution of connective and muscular structure.

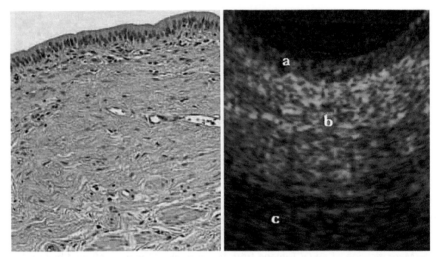

Fig. 7. Magnification of an OCT image from the normal MPD wall, confirmed by histology. From the surface of the duct, up to a depth of 1 mm, the following layers are recognizable: (a) the single layer of epithelial cells, approximately 0.04 to 0.08 mm thick, visible as a superficial, hyporeflective band; (b) the connective-fibro-muscular layer surrounding the epithelium, visible as a hyper-reflective layer approximately 0.36 to 0.56 mm thick; and (c) the connective and acinar structure close to the ductal wall epithelium, visible as a hyporeflective layer.

is visible until the working depth of penetration into the tissue of the near-focus probe (approximately 1 mm). Smooth muscle structure appears at OCT scanning as hyper-reflective, longitudinal strips within a context of hyporeflective tissue and is particularly recognizable at the level of SO.

Arteries, veins, and secondary pancreatic ducts are also identifiable by OCT, characterized by hypo- or nonreflective, well-delimited areas. Arteries show up as a brightly reflective intima enclosing a nonreflective area. Veins appear as larger than the arteries, with a thin, normo-reflective wall. Close to the MPD, OCT also shows some parts of accessory ducts, seen as nonreflective, well-delimited areas, larger than the vessels in diameter. Occasionally, during the OCT films acquisition, it was also possible to see the MPD communication.

The images acquired provide information on tissue architectural morphology that could have only previously been obtained with conventional biopsy. These results suggest that OCT could become a powerful imaging technology, enabling high-resolution diagnostic images to be obtained from the pancreatobiliary system during a diagnostic ERCP procedure.

OPTICAL COHERENCE TOMOGRAPHY RECOGNITION OF ABNORMAL, NON- NEOPLASTIC PANCREATICOBILIARY WALL STRUCTURE
Fibrotic Changes

OCT features concerning the fibrotic changes in the pancreaticobiliary wall structure regard only the intermediate layer of these structures, which corresponds in fact to the fibro-connective tissue, the only layer histologically involved in the fibrotic changes. The main characteristic of this alteration is the increased number of connective fibers of the intermediate layer that allow an increase in the thickness of the fibro-connective layer.

OCT investigation of these modifications shows an increase in the thickness of the intermediate layer and light backscattering. The inner layer, corresponding to the surface epithelium, and the outer, hyporeflective layer do not show significant differences from normal subjects. The three-layer architecture of the ductal wall is maintained and the boundary between the inner and intermediate layers appears still recognizable in all frames. Because of the increased reflectance of the intermediate layer, the boundary with the outer layer is generally more easily recognizable than in the normal subjects, although less regular (**Fig. 8**).

When the OCT probe is inserted across strictures in strict contact with the tissue surface, the ductal inner layer, corresponding to the superficial epithelium, may appear compressed and occasionally difficult to evaluate.

In a study performed by our group in patients with biliary type 1 sphincter of Oddi dysfunction (SOD)[27] the mean thickness of the inner, hyporeflective layer was 0.052 ± 0.007 mm (range 0.04–0.06 mm) and its reflectance was homogeneous; OCT findings did not differ in comparison with control subjects. Unlike in controls, OCT imaging in patients with SOD showed an increased thickness of the intermediate, hyper-reflective layer (mean 0.72 ± 0.028 mm - range 0.57–0.83 mm, versus 0.31 ± 0.014 mm - range 0.24–0.41 mm), with increased infrared light back-scattering, a sign of hyper-reflectance very likely caused by tissue fibrosis, as reported for the MPD wall in a previous study comparing OCT with histology, done in ex vivo specimens of chronic pancreatitis.[23] The intermediate layer in patients with SOD was 2.3 times thicker than in control patients (P<.0001) (**Fig. 9**).

OCT findings obtained in five patients by radial imaging from fibrotic strictures of the main pancreatic duct showed defined three-layer architecture of the wall, with a linear, regular surface, and different, homogeneous backscattering of the signal from each layer. However, in contrast with sphincter of Oddi ductal findings, the intermediate, connective-fibro-muscular layer was not significantly enlarged (0.3–0.55 mm thick) (**Fig. 10**).[12]

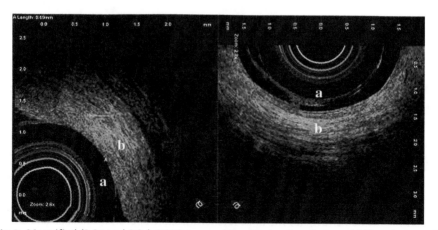

Fig. 8. Magnified (2.8x and 2.3x) OCT images of the SO structure in type 1 biliary SOD, with OCT probe maintained inside the ERCP catheter (a). The intermediate layer (b) appears markedly thickened, with increased infrared light back-scattering. Because of the marked hyper-reflectance of the intermediate layer, the boundary between it and the outer layer is generally more easily recognizable than in normal subjects.

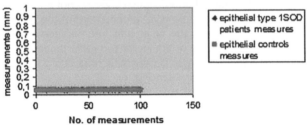

A   **Comparison of the OCT epithelial measures
between type 1 SOD patients and controls**

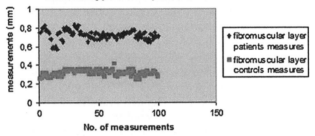

B   **Comparison of the OCT submucosal measures
between type 1 SOD patients and controls**

Fig. 9. Comparison of OCT epithelial and submucosal layers measures between patients with type 1 biliary SOD 1 and controls. (A) OCT epithelial layer thickness measurements in patients with type 1 SOD and controls. No significant difference was found between the two groups. (B) OCT subepithelial, fibro-muscular layer measurements in patients with type 1 SOD and controls. A significant difference (P < .0001) was found between the two groups.

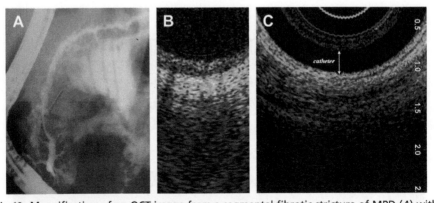

Fig. 10. Magnification of an OCT image from a segmental fibrotic stricture of MPD (A) with OCT probe outside (B) and inside (C) the ERCP catheter. (A) ERCP imaging of a segmental fibrotic stricture of MPD with OCT probe inserted into the stricture, identified by its radiopaque marker (*red arrow*). (B) The three-layer architecture appears maintained and differentiated. The inner, hyporeflective layer appears slightly larger than in the MPD of the normal pancreas. The intermediate layer appears more hyper-reflective than in normal tissue, probably because of a dense mononuclear cell infiltrate. (C) The inner hyporeflective layer is compressed by the ERCP catheter sheet (*white arrow*) and is not visible. This artifact renders the differential diagnosis with normal MPD wall substantially impossible.

Chronic Inflammatory Changes

In chronic inflammatory changes OCT still shows conserved three-layer architecture. An increased thickness with heterogeneous backscattering of the signal of the inner, epithelial layer and increased scattering in the periductal connective tissue (intermediate layer) were reported for inflammatory changes of the biliary tree in a few cases in a preliminary study.[26]

In an our ex-vivo study of main pancreatic duct in pancreatic surgical specimens, the inner, hyporeflective layer appeared slightly larger than normal (0.07–0.24 mm) and the intermediate layer appeared more hyper-reflective than in normal tissue (**Fig. 11**).[23] This is probably because of the dense mononuclear cell infiltrate related to inflammation. The backscattered signal was heterogeneous with marked hypo- or hyper-reflectance in some sections. However, the agreement between OCT and histology in the definition of MPD chronic inflammatory changes, in our experience, was poor (27.7%). In fact, we found no characteristic OCT patterns for inflammatory MPD changes, since the architecture of the layers and surface reflection was not substantially modified in normal and chronically inflamed epithelium.

OPTICAL COHERENCE TOMOGRAPHY RECOGNITION OF DYSPLASTIC AND NEOPLASTIC PANCREATICOBILIARY WALL STRUCTURE

Studies in vivo were performed in animals[24] and humans.[25] Disorganized layer architecture and altered backscattered light signal are the two main OCT features in patients with dysplastic and neoplastic changes. At present, the exact cause of the altered light scattering associated with dysplastic tissue by OCT imaging is unknown. A number of different factors have been suggested from different authors

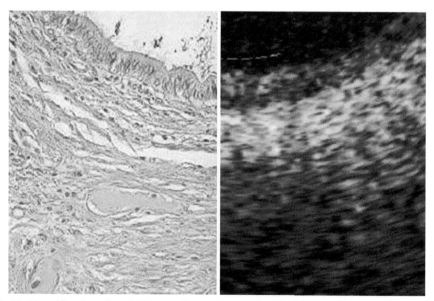

Fig. 11. Magnification of an OCT image from a MPD wall with chronic inflammatory changes, confirmed by histology. The three-layer architecture appears maintained and well differentiated. The inner, hyporeflective layer appears slightly larger than normal (0.07–0.24 mm). The intermediate layer appears more hyper-reflective than in normal tissue; this is probably because of the dense mononuclear cell infiltrate.

including: subcellular morphological changes; altered fibrovascular stroma and abnormal mucin content associated with neoplastic tissue change; and proliferation of cells leading to a loss of epithelial and stromal orientation and altered cytological features, such as an increased nuclear-to-cytoplasm ratio that may alter the infrared light back-scattering.[28] In its current form and resolution, OCT will likely localize areas displaying architectural distortion to guide biopsy.

Most of the studies published to date have used OCT imaging to detect dysplasia and early cancer within Barrett's epithelium. Since the penetration depth of OCT does not exceed 1to 2 mm, the technique could be useful not only in detecting dysplasia but also in staging superficial cancers that are difficult to stage accurately with ultrasound endoscopy. The technique appears, therefore, to be of crucial importance in the management of the disease.

Dysplastic and neoplastic MPD changes have been investigated by our group in humans in two ex vivo studies[6,23] performed on multiple surgical pancreatic specimens obtained from patients with pancreatic head adenocarcinoma. The OCT pattern in presence of dysplasia of the main pancreatic duct epithelium was characterized by an inner layer markedly thickened, strongly hyporeflective and heterogeneous; this OCT finding is probably caused by the initial structural disorganization (ie, increased mitosis and altered nucleus/cytoplasm ratio). The surface between the inner and intermediate layers appeared irregular. As in chronic inflammatory tissue, dysplasia also gave strong hyper-reflectance of the intermediate layer, particularly in the part closest to the inner layer. The outer layer did not differ from other nonmalignant conditions and appeared homogeneously hyporeflective (**Fig. 12**). However, in chronic pancreatitis and dysplasia only 62% of cases OCT and histology were concordant. K statistic used to assess agreement between the two procedures was equal to 0.059 for non-

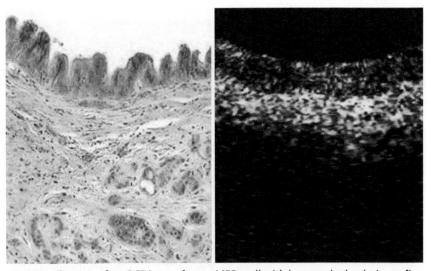

Fig.12. Magnification of an OCT image from a MPD wall with low-grade dysplasia confirmed by histology. The inner layer shows thickening (0.49 mm) and infrared light hyporeflectance, probably caused by the initial structural disorganization (increased mitosis and altered nucleus/cytoplasm ratio). The surface between the inner and intermediate layers appears irregular. As in chronic inflammatory tissue, dysplasia also gives strong hyper-reflectance of the intermediate layer, particularly in the part closest to the inner layer. The outer layer does not differ from other nonmalignant conditions and appears homogeneously hyporeflective.

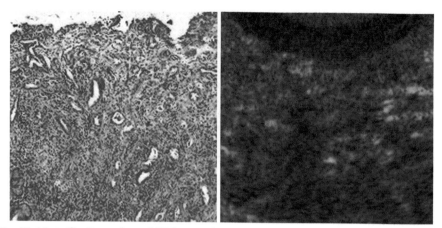

Fig. 13. Magnification of an OCT image from an adenocarcinoma-involved MPD wall, confirmed by histology. The wall architecture is totally subverted, with loss of the ductal parietal layers and unidentifiable connective-fibro-muscular layer and acinar tissue. The three layers and their linear, regular surface, normally giving a homogeneous back-scattered signal, are not recognizable. The OCT image has a heterogeneous back-scattered signal with minute, multiple, nonreflective areas in the disorganized pancreatic microstructure.

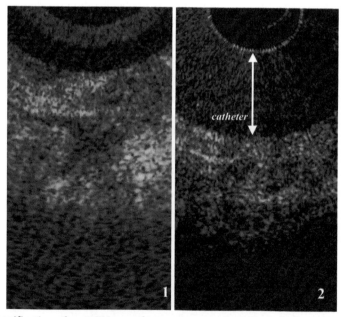

Fig. 14. Magnification of an OCT image from a segmental stricture of MPD in a patient with adenocarcinoma, with OCT probe outside (1) and inside (2) the ERCP catheter. (1) The wall architecture is totally subverted, with the loss of the ductal layer architecture; the three layers and their linear, regular surface, normally giving a homogeneous back-scattered signal are not recognizable. The OCT image has a heterogeneous back-scattered signal with minute, multiple, nonreflective areas in the disorganized pancreatic microstructure. (2) The totally subverted architecture is easily recognizable, even with the OCT probe inside the ERCP catheter (*white arrow*).

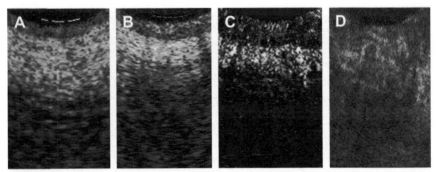

Fig. 15. Magnified OCT images from ex vivo sections of main pancreatic duct with normal tissue (*A*), chronic pancreatitis (*B*), low-grade dysplasia (*C*), and adenocarcinoma (*D*).

neoplastic MPD wall appearance. The same pattern is visualized for the biliary structures.

Overall, normal wall structure and chronic inflammatory or low-grade dysplastic changes cannot be distinguished in 38% of the sections because the architecture of the layers and surface-light reflection did not show a characteristic OCT pattern.

In the presence of pancreaticobiliary ductal adenocarcinoma, the wall architecture appears to be totally subverted at OCT imaging. The three layers of the ductal wall and their linear, regular surface, normally giving a homogeneous backscattered signal, are not recognizable. The margins between the connective-fibro-muscular layer and acinar tissue are unidentifiable. The backscattering of the signal appears strongly heterogeneous, with minute, multiple, nonreflective areas in the disorganized pancreatic microstructure (**Fig. 13**).

In an our ex vivo study all sections with histologically proven adenocarcinoma showed a totally subverted MPD wall architecture at OCT imaging, and in 100% of sections with adenocarcinoma OCT and histology were concordant (**Fig. 14**).[6]

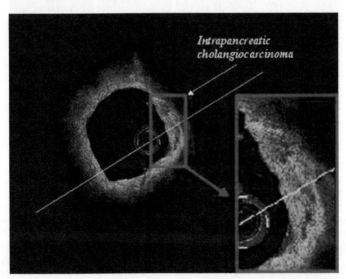

Fig. 16. Magnified OCT images of neoplastic tissue within the intrapancreatic portion of the common bile duct. The arrow indicates the enlargement of the red rectangular highlighted area of the neoplasia.

Table 1
Concordance of optical coherence tomography and brush cytology with final diagnosis in patients with non-neoplastic and neoplastic MPD strictures

	Final Diagnosis	
Technique	Non-neoplastic MPD Stricture	Neoplastic MPD Stricture
OCT	5/5	6/6
	100%	100%
Brush cytology	5/5	4/6
	100%	66.7%

Fig. 15 shows magnified OCT images from ex vivo sections of main pancreatic duct with normal tissue, chronic pancreatitis, low-grade dysplasia, and adenocarcinoma.

Totally subverted wall architecture was also observed by OCT in presence of neoplastic tissue within the common bile duct, described by our group in a report.[29] OCT imaging revealed a distorted CBD wall layer with heterogeneous light backscattering and an unrecognizable three-layer structure, suggesting a neoplastic lesion (**Fig. 16**).

We evaluated the diagnostic accuracy of OCT for the diagnosis of carcinoma, during ERCP, in a series of patients with MPD strictures of unknown etiology, considering that segmental strictures of the pancreas are sometimes difficult to investigate, particularly when they are located in the middle or in the tail of the gland. In these cases a definite diagnosis can be achieved only by cytology, either by intraductal brushing or fine needle aspiration biopsy (FNAB). In this study the accuracy of OCT for detection of neoplastic tissue was 100%, compared with 66.7 % for intraductal brush cytology. The study showed that OCT is feasible during an ERCP procedure and was superior to brush cytology in distinguishing non-neoplastic from neoplastic lesions (**Table 1**).[12]

SUMMARY

OCT appears to be a promising technique for real-time, high-resolution, cross-sectional imaging of the pancreaticobiliary ductal system, during the routinary pancreatobiliary endoscopy. The technique recognizes with high definition the surface epithelium and the surrounding connective-fibro-muscular tissue, and seems particularly useful in the differential diagnosis between non-neoplastic and neoplastic ductal lesions, given its superior resolution compared with other imaging modalities, such as EUS or catheter-probe EUS. Since OCT has a penetration depth that does not exceed 1.5 mm, it has a greater capability of diagnosing adenocarcinoma confined within epithelium and could therefore be useful in recognizing neoplastic ductal lesions at early stage.

Data obtained in clinical practice support the use of OCT imaging in the pancreaticobiliary ductal system to discriminate between non-neoplastic and neoplastic tissue when strictures of unknown etiology are identified during an ERCP procedure, being the diagnostic accuracy of OCT higher than reported for intraductal brush cytology. When OCT frames are obtained inside strictures, the ductal epithelial layer is generally compressed and can be visualized with difficulty through the transparent sheet of the ERCP catheter; better imaging can be obtained in these conditions by removing the ERCP catheter and leaving the OCT probe inside the stricture. The technique also seems promising for the evaluation of fibrotic changes, while its capability for recognition and definition of inflammatory changes remains poor.

Despite the promising studies reported in literature, with the current available OCT devices the recognition of dysplasia, mainly the differentiation between low- and high-grade dysplasia, appears difficult and further investigation is required.

At present, it seems to be fairly premature to affirm that OCT plays a role in the real-time diagnosis of dysplasia in vivo. However, improvements in axial and lateral resolutions to the subcellular level (<5 μm) together with the development of better light sources and optics, may allow dysplastic cells to be better identified in the future. Doppler OCT could also offer a unique ability to provide detailed subsurface imaging of mucosal microvascular networks. With expanding use in clinical practice and more experience in the interpretation of OCT imaging, we can expect more studies on the pancreaticobiliary ductal system, especially in presence of unknown strictures or precancerous and high-risk conditions, as primary sclerosing cholangitis awaiting liver transplantation.

REFERENCES

1. Huang D, Swanson EA, Lin CP, et al. Optical coherence tomography. Science 1991;254:1178–81.
2. Kobayashi K, Izatt JA, Kulkarni MD, et al. High-resolution cross-sectional imaging of the gastrointestinal tract using optical coherence tomography: preliminary results. Gastrointest Endosc 1998;47:515–23.
3. Cilesiz I, Fockens P, Kerindongo R, et al. Comparative optical coherence tomography imaging of human esophagus: how accurate is localization of the muscularis mucosae? Gastrointest Endosc 2002;56:852–7.
4. Testoni PA, Mariani A, Mangiavillano B, et al. Main pancreatic duct, common bile duct and sphincter of Oddi structure visualized by optical coherence tomography: an *ex vivo* study compared with histology. Dig Liver Dis 2006;38:409–14.
5. Tearney GJ, Brezinski ME, Southern JF, et al. Optical biopsy in human gastrointestinal tissue using optical coherence tomography. Am J Gastroenterol 1997; 92:1800–4.
6. Testoni PA, Mangiavillano B, Albarello L, et al. Optical coherence tomography to detect epithelial lesions of the main pancreatic duct: an *ex vivo* study. Am J Gastroenterol 2005;100:2777–83.
7. Pitris C, Jesser C, Boppart SA, et al. Feasibility of optical coherence tomography for high-resolution imaging of human gastrointestinal tract malignancies. J Gastroenterol 2000;35:87–92.
8. Sergeev AM, Gelikonov VM, Gelikonov GV, et al. In vivo endoscopic OCT imaging of precancer and cancer states of human mucosa. Opt Express 1997;1:432–40.
9. Tearney GJ, Brezinski ME, Bouma BE, et al. In vivo endoscopic optical biopsy with optical coherence tomography. Science 1997;276:2037–9.
10. Pfau PR, Sivak MV Jr, Chak A, et al. Criteria for the diagnosis of dysplasia by endoscopic optical coherence tomography. Gastrointest Endosc 2003;58: 196–202.
11. Isenberg G, Sivak MV Jr, Chak A, et al. Accuracy of endoscopic optical coherence tomography in the detection of dysplasia in Barrett' esophagus: a prospective, double-blinded study. Gastrointest Endosc 2005;62:825–31.
12. Testoni PA, Mariani A, Mangiavillano B, et al. Intraductal optical coherence tomography for investigating main pancreatic duct strictures. Am J Gastroenterol 2007;102:269–74.
13. Swanson EA, Izatt JA, Hee MR, et al. In vivo retinal imaging by optical coherence tomography. Opt Lett 1993;18:1864–6.

14. Fujimoto JG. Optical coherence tomography for ultrahigh resolution in vivo imaging. Nat Biotechnol 2003;21:1361–7.
15. Swanson EA. High-speed optical coherence domain reflectometry. Opt Lett 1992; 17:151–3.
16. Das A, Sivak MV, Chak A, et al. High-resolution endoscopic imaging of the GI tract: a comparative study of optical coherence tomography versus high-frequency catheter probe EUS. Gastrointest Endosc 2001;54:219–24.
17. Sivak MV, Kobayashi K, Izatt JA, et al. High-resolution endoscopic imaging of the GI tract using optical coherence tomography. Gastrointest Endosc 2000;51: 474–9.
18. Shen B, Zuccaro G Jr. Optical coherence tomography in the gastrointestinal tract. Gastrointest Endosc Clin N Am 2004;14:555–71.
19. Zuccaro G, Gladkova N, Vargo J, et al. Optical coherence tomography of the esophagus and proximal stomach in health and disease. Am J Gastroenterol 2001;96:2633–9.
20. Bouma BE, Tearney GJ, Compton CC, et al. High-resolution imaging of the human esophagus and stomach in vivo using optical coherence tomography. Gastrointest Endosc 2000;51:467–74.
21. Poneros JM, Brand S, Bouma BE, et al. A diagnosis of specialized intestinal metaplasia by optical coherence tomography. Gastroenterology 2001;120:7–12.
22. Tearney GJ, Brezinski ME, Southern JF, et al. Optical biopsy in human pancreatobiliary tissue using optical coherence tomography. Dig Dis Sci 1998;43:1193–9.
23. Testoni PA, Mangiavillano B, Albarello L, et al. Optical coherence tomography compared with histology of the main pancreatic duct structure in normal and pathological conditions: an ex vivo study. Dig Liver Dis 2006;38:688–95.
24. Singh P, Chak A, Willis JE, et al. In vivo optical coherence tomography imaging of the pancreatic and biliary ductal system. Gastrointest Endosc 2005;62:970.
25. Poneros JM, Tearney GJ, Shiskov M, et al. Optical coherence tomography of the biliary tree during ERCP. Gastrointest Endosc 2002;55:84–8.
26. Seitz U, Freund J, Jaeckle S, et al. First in vivo optical coherence tomography in the human bile duct. Endoscopy 2001;33:1018–21.
27. Testoni PA, Mangiavillano B, Mariani A, et al. Investigation of Oddi sphincter structure by optical coherence tomography in patients with biliary-type 1 dysfunction: A pilot in vivo study. Dig Liver Dis 2009;27 [Epub ahead of print].
28. Jaekle S, Gladkova N, Feldchtein F, et al. In vivo endoscopic optical coherence tomography of esophagitis, Barrett's esophagus, and adenocarcinoma of the esophagus. Endoscopy 2000;32:750–5.
29. Mangiavillano B, Mariani A, Petrone MC. An intrapancreatic cholangiocarcinoma detected with optical coherence tomography during ERCP. Clin Gastroenterol Hepatol 2008;6:A30.

Index

Note: Page numbers of article titles are in **boldface** type.

Gastrointest Endoscopy Clin N Am 19 (2009) 655–660
doi:10.1016/S1052-5157(09)00120-2
1052-5157/09/$ – see front matter © 2009 Elsevier Inc. All rights reserved.

giendo.theclinics.com

United States Postal Service
Statement of Ownership, Management, and Circulation
(All Periodicals Publications Except Requestor Publications)

1. Publication Title	2. Publication Number	3. Filing Date
Gastrointestinal Endoscopy Clinics of North America	0 1 2 - 6 0 0 3	9/15/09

4. Issue Frequency	5. Number of Issues Published Annually	6. Annual Subscription Price
Jan, Apr, Jul, Oct	4	$259.00

7. Complete Mailing Address of Known Office of Publication (Not printer) (Street, city, county, state, and ZIP+4®)

Elsevier Inc.
360 Park Avenue South
New York, NY 10010-1710

Contact Person
Stephen Bushing
Telephone (Include area code)
215-239-3688

8. Complete Mailing Address of Headquarters or General Business Office of Publisher (Not printer)

Elsevier Inc., 360 Park Avenue South, New York, NY 10010-1710

9. Full Names and Complete Mailing Addresses of Publisher, Editor, and Managing Editor (Do not leave blank)

Publisher (Name and complete mailing address)

John Schrefer, Elsevier, Inc., 1600 John F. Kennedy Blvd. Suite 1800, Philadelphia, PA 19103-2899

Editor (Name and complete mailing address)

Kerry Holland, Elsevier, Inc., 1600 John F. Kennedy Blvd. Suite 1800, Philadelphia, PA 19103-2899

Managing Editor (Name and complete mailing address)

Catherine Bewick, Elsevier, Inc., 1600 John F. Kennedy Blvd. Suite 1800, Philadelphia, PA 19103-2899

10. Owner (Do not leave blank. If the publication is owned by a corporation, give the name and address of the corporation immediately followed by the names and addresses of all stockholders owning or holding 1 percent or more of the total amount of stock. If not owned by a corporation, give the names and addresses of the individual owners. If owned by a partnership or other unincorporated firm, give its name and address as well as those of each individual owner. If the publication is published by a nonprofit organization, give its name and address.)

Full Name	Complete Mailing Address
Wholly owned subsidiary of	4520 East-West Highway
Reed/Elsevier, US holdings	Bethesda, MD 20814

11. Known Bondholders, Mortgagees, and Other Security Holders Owning or Holding 1 Percent or More of Total Amount of Bonds, Mortgages, or Other Securities. If none, check box ☐ None

Full Name	Complete Mailing Address
N/A	

12. Tax Status (For completion by nonprofit organizations authorized to mail at nonprofit rates) (Check one)
The purpose, function, and nonprofit status of this organization and the exempt status for federal income tax purposes:
☐ Has Not Changed During Preceding 12 Months
☐ Has Changed During Preceding 12 Months (Publisher must submit explanation of change with this statement)

PS Form 3526, September 2007 (Page 1 of 3 (Instructions Page 3)) PSN 7530-01-000-9931 PRIVACY NOTICE: See our Privacy policy in www.usps.com

---

13. Publication Title			14. Issue Date for Circulation Data Below
Gastrointestinal Endoscopy Clinics of North America			April 2009

15. Extent and Nature of Circulation			Average No. Copies Each Issue During Preceding 12 Months	No. Copies of Single Issue Published Nearest to Filing Date
a. Total Number of Copies (Net press run)			1297	1088
b. Paid Circulation (By Mail and Outside the Mail)	(1)	Mailed Outside-County Paid Subscriptions Stated on PS Form 3541. (Include paid distribution above nominal rate, advertiser's proof copies, and exchange copies)	497	416
	(2)	Mailed In-County Paid Subscriptions Stated on PS Form 3541 (Include paid distribution above nominal rate, advertiser's proof copies, and exchange copies)		
	(3)	Paid Distribution Outside the Mails Including Sales Through Dealers and Carriers, Street Vendors, Counter Sales, and Other Paid Distribution Outside USPS®	210	167
	(4)	Paid Distribution by Other Classes Mailed Through the USPS (e.g. First-Class Mail®)		
c. Total Paid Distribution (Sum of 15b (1), (2), (3), and (4))			707	583
d. Free or Nominal Rate Distribution (By Mail and Outside the Mail)	(1)	Free or Nominal Rate Outside-County Copies Included on PS Form 3541	93	83
	(2)	Free or Nominal Rate In-County Copies Included on PS Form 3541		
	(3)	Free or Nominal Rate Copies Mailed at Other Classes Through the USPS (e.g. First-Class Mail)		
	(4)	Free or Nominal Rate Distribution Outside the Mail (Carriers or other means)		
e. Total Free or Nominal Rate Distribution (Sum of 15d (1), (2), (3) and (4))			93	83
f. Total Distribution (Sum of 15c and 15e)			800	666
g. Copies not Distributed (See instructions to publishers #4 (page #3))			497	422
h. Total (Sum of 15f and g)			1297	1088
i. Percent Paid (15c divided by 15f times 100)			88.38%	87.54%

16. Publication of Statement of Ownership
☐ If the publication is a general publication, publication of this statement is required. Will be printed in the October 2009 issue of this publication. ☐ Publication not required

17. Signature and Title of Editor, Publisher, Business Manager, or Owner

Stephen R. Bushing — Date S-eptember 15, 2009
Stephen R. Bushing – Subscription Services Coordinator
I certify that all information furnished on this form is true and complete. I understand that anyone who furnishes false or misleading information on this form or who omits material or information requested on the form may be subject to criminal sanctions (including fines and imprisonment) and/or civil sanctions (including civil penalties).

PS Form 3526, September 2007 (Page 2 of 3)

Moving?

Make sure your subscription moves with you!

To notify us of your new address, find your **Clinics Account Number** (located on your mailing label above your name), and contact customer service at:

Email: journalscustomerservice-usa@elsevier.com

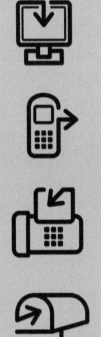

800-654-2452 (subscribers in the U.S. & Canada)
314-447-8871 (subscribers outside of the U.S. & Canada)

Fax number: 314-447-8029

Elsevier Health Sciences Division
Subscription Customer Service
3251 Riverport Lane
Maryland Heights, MO 63043

*To ensure uninterrupted delivery of your subscription, please notify us at least 4 weeks in advance of move.

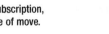

Printed and bound by CPI Group (UK) Ltd, Croydon, CR0 4YY

03/10/2024

01040443-0017